Vestibular Processing
Dysfunction
in Children

Vestibular Processing Dysfunction in Children

Kenneth J. Ottenbacher and Margaret A. Short
Editors

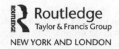

Routledge
Taylor & Francis Group

NEW YORK AND LONDON

First Published by

The Haworth Press, Inc., 28 East 22 Street, New York, NY 10010

Transferred to Digital Printing 2009 by Routledge
270 Madison Ave, New York NY 10016
2 Park Square, Milton Park, Abingdon, Oxon, OX14 4RN

Vestibular Processing Dysfunction in Children has also been published as *Physical & Occupational Therapy in Pediatrics*, Volume 5, Numbers 2/3, Summer/Fall 1985.

Library of Congress Cataloging in Publication Data
Main entry under title:

Vestibular processing dysfunction in children.

　　Published also as Physical & occupational therapy in pediatrics, v. 5, no. 2/3, summer/fall 1985.
　　Includes bibliographies.
　　1. Vestibular apparatus—Diseases. 2. Vestibular function tests. 3. Pediatric otolaryngology. I. Ottenbacher, Kenneth J. II. Short, Margaret A.
[DNLM: 1. Labyrinth Diseases—in infancy & childhood. 2. Vestibular Apparatus—physiopathology.
W1 PH683P v. 5 no. 2/3 / WV 255 V5835]
RF260.V47　　　1985　　　618.92'097882　　　85-8636
ISBN 0-86656-431-4
ISBN 0-86656-432-2 (pbk.)

Publisher's Note
The publisher has gone to great lengths to ensure the quality of this reprint but points out that some imperfections in the original may be apparent.

Vestibular Processing Dysfunction in Children

Physical & Occupational Therapy in Pediatrics
Volume 5, Numbers 2/3

CONTENTS

**Vestibular Stimulation as Early Experience:
Historical Perspectives and Research Implications** 135
Margaret A. Short, PhD, OTR

MARTHA C. PIPER, PhD, *Associate Professor and Director, School of Physical and Occupational Therapy, McGill University, Montreal, Quebec, Canada*

DONALD K. ROUTH, PhD, *Professor, Department of Psychology, The University of Iowa*

JOHN P. SCHOLZ, MA, LPT, *Research Assistant, Haskins Laboratories, New Haven, CT*

MARGARET A. SHORT, PhD, OTR, *Saratoga Springs, NY*

EARL SIEGEL, MD, *Professor of Maternal and Child Health and Clinical Professor of Pediatrics, University of North Carolina at Chapel Hill*

JOYCE W. SPARLING, MS, LPT, OTR, *Doctoral Candidate, Division of Special Education, School of Education, University of North Carolina at Chapel Hill*

NAPOLEON WOLANSKI, PhD, DSc, *Head, Department of Human Ecology of the Polish Academy of Sciences, Warsaw, Poland*

MARILYN SEIF WORKINGER, MS, *Speech-Language Pathologist, Marshfield Clinic, Marshfield, WI*

JANET E. YOUNG, MD, RPT, *Chief, Developmental Pediatrics, Fitzsimons Army Medical Center, Aurora, CO*

Vestibular Processing Dysfunction in Children

MESSAGE FROM THE EDITORS

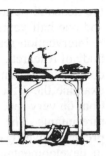

A well-developed body of research with both clinical and theoretical implications should include a variety of studies contributed by individuals from different backgrounds, and with diverse orientations. Such a body of research literature should contain anatomical investigations, analyses of instruments designed to clinically assess specific functions, descriptive behavioral studies, intervention research, literature reviews, and finally, analyses which place the existing research within the broader context of scientific literature. As editors of this special edition of *Physical and Occupational Therapy in Pediatrics,* we have assembled such a collection of articles.

The first article in this volume is a comprehensive examination of the structure of the vestibular system. Written by David Clark, an experienced anatomist and researcher in the study of the clinical effects of vestibular stimulation, this study provides a strong foundation for viewing the enormous complexity and interactions of the vestibular system. Patricia Montgomery's analytical review of vestibular-related assessment procedures provides a logical link between Clark's anatomical study and the clinical manifestations of vestibular-processing functions.

One specific vestibular-related measure of clinical interest to therapists is the *Southern California Postrotary Nystagmus Test* (SCPNT). This instrument is widely used by researchers and therapists exploring vestibular-related functions. Rebecca Dutton provides readers with an examination of the SCPNT. Following Dutton's detailed account of the SCPNT, Jean Deitz and Terry Crowe demonstrate the clinical relevance of this test. Deitz and Crowe's article is another important addition to their already comprehensive research into the clinical significance of postrotary nystagmus measures in pre-school children. In this volume, they describe the relationship among visual-motor, gross motor and cognitive developmental characteristics of children who were classified high-risk during the neonatal period, and who exhibit zero postrotary nystagmus at four and one-half years of age.

Intervention research is an important component of a well-developed body of research. Two studies in this collection provide examples of well-controlled, systematic intervention studies. Pelletier, Short and Nelson examine the effects of a vestibular-related intervention, waterbed flotation, on very specific, well-delineated motor behaviors of healthy premature infants. The study conducted by Lydic and colleagues is based on previous investigations of controlled rotation on the motor performance of developmentally delayed infants. In both of these investigations the relationship between a vestibular-related intervention and motor behavior is examined, a relationship well-documented in previous theories and experimentation. Both studies provide strict experimental criteria and thorough operational definitions for the selection of subject populations, yet each of these studies also provides a unique approach to vestibular-related stimulation. Pelletier and associates examine premature infant motor behaviors within the theoretical and clinical context of approach-avoidance behavior, and Lydic and colleagues provide important clinical data regarding the use of two different development instruments in measuring motor abilities of delayed, hypotonic infants.

This special volume contributes to the expanding body of vestibular-related clinical research by providing two analytical reviews. Ottenbacher and Petersen use meta-analysis to review and organize a large body of research, giving much needed generalizations regarding the clinical efficacy of vestibular stimulation. The analysis provides valuable suggestions for the selection of dependent variables in subsequent studies. It also provides a clinical model for understanding the methods and utility of quantitatively synthesizing research literature.

The second review article by Short provides readers with a general overview and summary. The article is important because it places literature related to vestibular stimulation in the much broader context of early experience. Short examines vestibular stimulation research as it has changed over the past several decades, and makes predictions regarding future directions for clinical research in this area. She also discusses changing perspectives regarding infancy and development and how current trends exploring interactionism and human ecology will affect the way we conduct clinical research and apply the findings and information to our clinical practice.

In summary, this collection of articles is intended to help expand, organize, and enhance our understanding of the scientific and clinical relevance of vestibular-related research. While we believe this collection presents important information, it should not be perceived as definitive.

Instead, we hope that these articles will serve to initiate more questions, to stimulate more investigation, and ultimately, to promote more effective treatment procedures for the consumers of our therapeutic services.

Kenneth J. Ottenbacher, PhD, OTR
Margaret A. Short, PhD, OTR
Guest Editors

The Vestibular System: An Overview of Structure and Function

David L. Clark, PhD

INTRODUCTION

The vestibular system is phylogenetically old and has neuroanatomical connections with many other systems, both motor and sensory. Some basic physiological interactions of the vestibular system with other systems are partially understood; however, the full impact of vestibular input on central nervous system (CNS) function is not known.

This chapter is limited to basic anatomy and physiology of some of the better understood portions of the vestibular system. The sensory end organ in the inner ear functions as a transducer of vestibular-appropriate sensory stimuli. The vestibular nuclear complex consists of a number of nuclei and cell groups, but only the four major nuclei are discussed. Portions of the cerebellum, some of which receive primary vestibular afferents, also are involved in vestibular reflexes. Descending vestibular activity is discussed in terms of the vestibulospinal and reticulospinal tracts which appear to share in controlling many postural reflexes. Long descending pathways apparently are more responsive to otolith rather than to semicircular canal input. Ascending pathways play a major role in controlling eye movements in response to movements of the head. Ascending pathways primarily reflect semicircular canal signals, with some otolith influence. Since the vestibular input functions to help maintain a stable retinal image, visual feedback and the cerebellum are important factors in the vestibulo-ocular reflex.

END ORGAN

The ear may be divided into three parts: (1) the outer ear, (2) the middle ear, and (3) the inner ear. The outer ear consists of the pinna and the external auditory canal which terminates medially at the tympanic membrane. The middle ear is an air-filled cavity containing the ossicles which

David L. Clark is an Associate Professor, Department of Anatomy, College of Medicine, Ohio State University, Columbus, OH 43210.

conduct auditory vibrations from the tympanic membrane to the inner ear. The external and middle ears are concerned only with hearing, but the inner ear functions for both hearing and equilibrium. The inner ear is made up of a series of fluid-filled chambers and ducts (Figure 1). One fluid-filled space lies within the other. The outer space is the perilymphatic space while the inner space is the endolymphatic space. The perilymphatic space is filled with a fluid called perilymph, and the endolymphatic space is filled with endolymph. The tissue surrounding the perilymphatic space is part of the temporal bone. Embryologically, the cartilagenous precursor of the bone tissue forms a capsule immediately around the perilymphatic space and this tissue is called the osseous labyrinth.[1] The thin membrane separating the perilymphatic space from the endolymphatic space is the membranous labyrinth. The neuroepithelium for the auditory and vestibular portions of the ear is found within the endolymphatic space.

The vestibular portion of the ear has three parts: (1) the utricle, (2) the saccule, and (3) the semicircular canals. The utricle and saccule lie just medial and posterior to the cochlea, or auditory portion of the ear. The endolymph of the utricle and saccule is continuous with that of the semicircular canals and of the scala media of the cochlea. The utricle and saccule are almost identical, both anatomically and physiologically, and are often collectively referred to as the otolith organ. The term otolith ("ear stone") refers to thousands of calcium carbonate crystals (otolithic or statolithic crystals) which are imbedded in the surface of the epithelium of these two sensory organs. The neuroepithelium of the otolith organ, including otolithic crystals, is called the macula.

Each ear contains three semicircular canals. Each is paired with

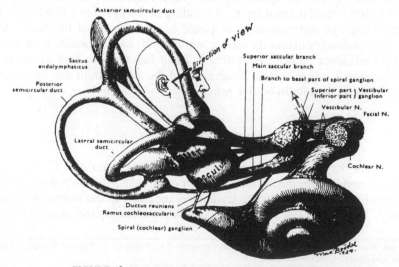

FIGURE 1[2]. The endolymph-filled membranous labyrinth.

another canal in the opposite ear. The membranous semicircular canals consist of an endolymph-filled duct and ampulla. The duct is curved and forms the "semicircle". It opens at one end into the utricle and the other end joins with its ampulla. The ampulla contains the neuroepithelium: the crista ampullaris. The crista ampullaris, is in many ways, similar to the macula of the otolith organ.

The structure of both the otolith and semicircular canal neuroepithelium is basically the same. The neuroepithelium consists of sensory hair cells, supportive cells, nerve fibers, nerve endings and superstructural elements such as the cupula and otolithic crystals, which can be considered to function as mechanical transducers to transform angular and linear acceleration into pattern-specific afferent nerve signals.

Two types of vestibular sensory hair cells have been identified (Figure 2). The Type II hair cell is phylogenetically more primitive and its cell body takes on a columnar appearance. The peripheral processes of several afferent neurons make direct synaptic contact with the Type II hair cell surface. The Type I hair cell has a light-bulb shape, and a peripheral afferent process forms an expanded envelope, or calyx, that intimately envelops the surface of the hair cell. Efferent fibers also interact with both hair cell types. Efferent fibers terminate directly upon the body of cell Type II, thus forming a synapse peripheral to the hair cell-afferent synapse. Efferent fibers to the Type I cell, however, make contact with the afferent calyx, not the surface of the Type I hair cell.

Cilia project from the surface of the cuticular plate of each hair cell. From 60 to 100 stereocilia but only one kinocilium project from the surface of each hair cell. The stereocilia are homogenous in cross-section, are rather stiff and are anchored with small rootlets which penetrate through the cuticle. The kinocilium is longer than the longest stereocilium and is found on one side of the bundle of stereocilia. The asymmetry produced by the location of the kinocilium produces a polarization of each hair cell. In the crista of the horizontal semicircular canal, the kinocilium of each hair cell is located on the utricular side of the ampulla, that is, toward the midline; therefore, the polarity of each hair cell is extended to provide polarity of each crista ampullaris. The polarity is reversed in the vertical canal cristae. In the cristae of the vertical canals, the kinocilia are all located on the distal pole of the hair cells, toward the semicircular canal duct.[4]

Electrophysiological experiments on the semicircular canals show the consequence of the anatomical polarity.[5,6] In a majority of units sampled, spontaneous activity was found when the cupula was in the resting position (Figure 3). When the cupula was deflected in the direction of the kinocilium, the rate of discharge increased. When deflected in the direction away from the kinocilium, the level of spontaneous activity decreased.

The polarization of hair cells of the macula of the utricle and saccule

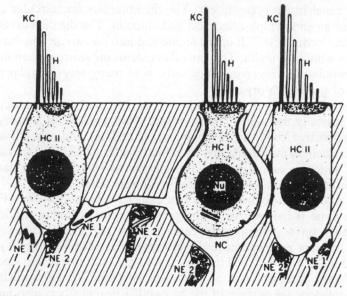

FIGURE 2[3]. Schematic diagram of the vestibular neuroepithelial hair cell Type I (HCI) and hair cell Type II (HCII) with sensory endings (NE1) on hair cell Type II and afferent calyx (NC) on hair cell Type I. Efferent terminals (NE2) are shown synapsing on both hair cell surfaces and on afferent fibers. Nu, nucleus; KC, kinocilium; H, stereocilia.

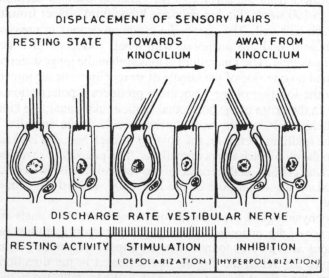

FIGURE 3[4]. Primary ampullary afferents show spontaneous discharge while the cupula is in a resting condition (left). If cupula deflection deflects the cilia toward the kinocilia, discharge rate increases (middle). When deflected away from the kinocilia, the discharge rate decreases (right).

is more complex. Hair cells in any one area of the macula tend to be oriented in the same direction; however, over the entire surface a changing pattern of polarization is seen. Over the surface of the utricular macula, directionality dictated by the kinocilia forms a laterally directed, fan-like pattern beginning at the medial edge up to a curved boundary line which passes near the center of the macula (Figure 4). Lateral to the boundary line, kinocilia are medially directed.

A different pattern exists on the macula of the saccule (Figure 5). A curving boundary line courses from superior to inferior across the surface; however, the kinocilia do not face each other across the boundary line as in the utricle, but face away from each other. In the case of both maculae, the boundary line tends to coincide with the striola where smaller otolithic crystals are found. The small crystals coupled with the opposing polarity along the boundary line suggest a specialized region of the macula.[8]

The neuroepithelium, or macula, of the otolith organ consists of a single layer of neurosensory hair cells interspersed with supporting cells, all on a basement membrane. Cilia project from the surface of each neurosensory hair cell and project into a gelatinous substance which lies as a layer above the neurosensory and supporting cells. The otolithic crystals form the most superficial layer of the macula. The otolith crystals are imbedded in the surface of the gelatinous substance and apparently are covered with some kind of adhesive which keeps them from breaking away from each other and from the gelatinous substance.

The otolith organ functions to detect linear acceleration. Linear acceleration is a change in linear velocity, and is experienced, for example,

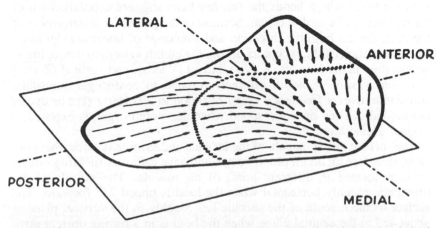

FIGURE 4[7]. The plane of the surface of the utricle approximates the horizontal plane when the head is tipped forward 25°. The anterior third of the surface is raised slightly. The arrows indicate the direction of polarization dictated by the location of kinocilia.

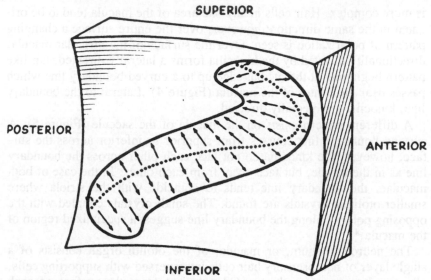

FIGURE 5[7]. The plane of the surface of the saccule is approximately vertical. The surface is slightly concave, and the kinocilia are oriented away from a curving centerline as indicated by the arrows.

when your car accelerates away from a stoplight, or decelerates at a stop sign. Linear acceleration is also experienced as we go up or down in an elevator. In fact, since gravity is a form of linear acceleration, the otolith organ is sensitive to sustained head tilt in any position. Linear acceleration is detected because the otolithic crystals are more dense than the endolymph fluid or the gelatinous layer in which they are imbedded. A shearing force which bends the sensory hairs triggers depolarization of the hair cells. The otolith organ, because of the patterned arrangement of the cilia, detects both the direction and amplitude of linear acceleration. The distribution of the receptors allows the otolith system to detect linear acceleration in the fore-aft (X axis), lateral (Y axis), and vertical (Z axis) directions. Primary otolith afferents respond to centrifugal sinusoidal stimulation over a frequency range of 0.006 to 2.0 Hertz (Hz or cycles per second).[9] They do not respond when the otolith organ is exposed to angular acceleration.[10]

The surface of the macula of the utricule and saccule is somewhat concave, therefore an acceleration vector will have different shearing effects on cells located in different areas of the macula. The macula of the utricule is roughly horizontal when the head is tipped 25° forward. The surface of the macula of the saccule lies roughly in the vertical plane at about 45° to the sagittal plane when the head is in a resting upright position.

The neuroepithelium, or crista ampullaris, of the semicircular canal, is made up of a single layer of a mixture of neurosensory and supporting cells. Both Type I and Type II neurosensory cells are included and each neurosensory cell has many stereocilia and a single kinocilium which project into a gelatinous layer, in a manner similar to that of the macula. Here the similarity ends. The crista contains no crystals, and the gelatinous layer, which contains the cilia, is thicker.

The gelatinous layer of the crista ampullaris is called the cupula. The cupula extends across the lumen of the ampulla of the semicircular canal and may be lightly attached to the wall on the opposite side. The cupula is of the same density and viscosity as the endolymph which surrounds it; therefore, unlike the macula, the cupula and semicircular canal are insensitive to linear acceleration and gravity.[10] The cupula, however, is sensitive to any movement of the endolymph fluid on either side of it. Since the semicircular canals form a complete ring with the help of the cavity of the utricle which completes the circle, head movements in a circular direction are sensed by the semicircular canals. Specifically, the semicircular canals are sensitive to angular acceleration. Angular acceleration is a change in angular velocity, that is, a change in the rate at which the head is turning. We measure angular velocity in revolutions per minute (rpm) or more often in degrees per second (°/sec).

The three semicircular canals of each ear lie in different planes of space. Actually, we should speak of the canals as pairs as they function together with one of the pair being in the left ear and the other of the pair being in the right ear. The horizontal semicircular canal lies almost in the horizontal plane. The anterior portion of the paired horizontal canals is about 30° higher than the posterior portion when the head is in approximately the normal, upright, resting position. In order to place the horizontal canals into the horizontal plane, we would tip the nose downward 30° (Figure 6).

The other pairs of semicircular canals lie in the vertical plane. The right anterior canal lies in the same vertical plane as does the left posterior canal. In order to place these two canals into the earth horizontal plane, we need to tip the head as far to the right as possible (90°), then turn the head to look upward, about 45° (Figure 7). The left anterior and right posterior canals lie in the same vertical plane, but this vertical plane is 90° to the vertical plane coincident with the other two vertical canals. In order to place this last set of vertical canals in the earth horizontal, we would need to tip the head to the left 90°, then turn the head to look upward about 45°.

A common form of angular acceleration used to stimulate the semicircular canals in therapy or in testing is an impulsive change in angular velocity. This may be defined as a change in angular velocity requiring less than one second. The magnitude of deflection of the cupula resulting from such a change in angular velocity is dependent upon the angular

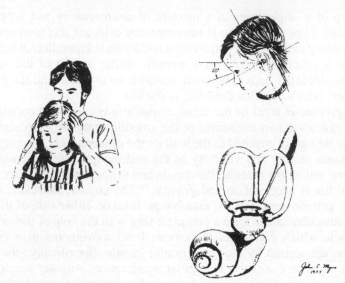

FIGURE 6. The plane of the horizontal semicircular canals approximates the earth horizontal when the head is tipped forward about 30°. A convenient indicator is an imaginary line between the external auditory meatus and lateral canthus of the eye. Since this plane is raised anteriorly approximately 10°, dropping this plane 20° below earth horizontal will depress the horizontal canals about 30°.

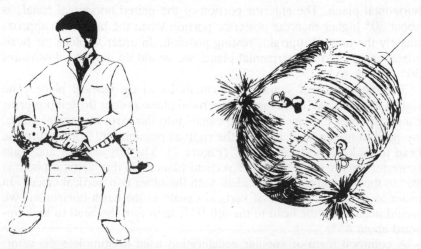

FIGURE 7. The vertical semicircular canals lie in the vertical plane. The paired right anterior and left posterior canals are at right angles to the paired left anterior and right posterior canals. The girl's head viewed from above shows that while held in the therapist's lap, the right anterior and left posterior canals are in the earth horizontal plane. Rotation about the therapist's vertical axis, as in a rotary chair, will stimulate the canals lying in the plane of rotation.

velocity before and after the brief episode of acceleration (deceleration). Once an impulse of angular acceleration has been experienced and the cupula is deflected, some time is required for the cupula to return to its resting position. The rate at which the cupula returns is described as the "time constant" of cupular return. Another form of stimulation is a series of sinusoidal angular head movements. Semicircular canal afferents respond in a linear fashion in a range from about 0.01 to 7 Hz. This range overlaps that of the otolith organ but extends into higher frequency range.

The semicircular canal with its cupula has been described as a highly overdamped torsion pendulum.[11] During head angular acceleration, as the head begins to turn, the endolymph and the cupula tend to remain stationary because of the inertia of the cupula-endolymph. As the head accelerates, the cupula deflects proportional to the instantaneous angular velocity of the head. The firing pattern transferred by the ampullary nerve to the vestibular nuclei reflects the degree of cupular deflection; therefore, because of the mechanics of the canal, the neurophysiological signal is a measure of head angular velocity. The stimulus, angular acceleration, is represented by the neurophysiological signal in the ampullary nerve as an integrated signal, angular velocity. Once angular acceleration ceases, the signal decays since the cupula, because of its inherent springiness, returns like a pendulum to its resting position. It returns slowly and does not overshoot its resting position, therefore acting in an overdamped manner.

If a person is rotated at a constant angular velocity for a period of a minute or so, then impulsively stopped, we can see a back and forth shimmering of the eyes of the test subject. This eye movement is called nystagmus. Nystagmus is made up of a slow component (slow phase) and a fast component (fast phase). The fast phase resets the eye rapidly (up to about 700 °/sec)[12] so that a subsequent slow phase eye movement can take place. The speed of a slow phase eye movement is greatest immediately following an impulsive deceleration and may reach 150 °/sec. The slow phase is dependent upon the vestibular system. The anatomical substrate of the fast phase is not well understood but does not directly involve the vestibular system.

The afferent terminals that make synaptic contact with the hair cells of the macula and crista ampullaris are the peripheral processes of the cell bodies of the vestibular division of the statoacoustic or eighth cranial nerve. The cell bodies are bipolar in shape and collectively make up the vestibular ganglion (of Scarpa) located in the internal auditory meatus. The vestibular nerve, after leaving the ganglion, enters the brainstem at the cerebellopontine angle where the fibers branch into ascending and longer descending branches. Some of these primary afferent fibers continue directly to the ipsilateral cerebellum where they terminate as mossy fibers, primarily in the cortex of the nodulus, uvula and flocculus. The majority of the primary afferent fibers terminate in the ipsilateral vestibular nuclear complex. None cross to the vestibular nuclei of the opposite side.

VESTIBULAR NUCLEI

The vestibular nuclear complex makes up a large portion of the dorso-lateral brainstem in the region of the pontomedullary junction. It consists of four major vestibular nuclei and a number of smaller accessory nuclei. The major inputs to these nuclei arise from the following sources: primary afferent fibers from vestibular receptors, the reticular formation, and the cerebellum which comprises the largest component.

The superior vestibular nucleus (SVN) is the most rostral of the main nuclei. It is made up of cells of various sizes. Primary afferent fibers, largely from the vertical semicircular canals, terminate in the central region of the SVN, where its larger cells are concentrated.[13] Horizontal canal units and otolith-sensitive cells are present, but fewer in number than vertical canal units. Fibers from the cerebellar fastigial nucleus tend to terminate in the peripheral part of the SVN. Cells from all areas of the nucleus give rise to fibers that ascend in the brain stem. The SVN also has extensive commissural connections with the contralateral SVN.

The lateral vestibular nucleus (LVN) lies ventral to SVN and lateral to the medial vestibular nucleus (MVN). LVN is frequently called Deiters' nucleus in reference to the giant cells of Deiters found here. The LVN also contains many smaller neurons, the giant cells being more abundant in the caudal portion of the nucleus. The LVN receives a modest number of primary afferents from the labyrinth, and their termination is restricted to the ventral part of the nucleus. The majority of these primary fibers are from the otolith organs.[14] Commissural fibers are reported to be absent in the LVN.[15] Cells of the LVN have a specific and important relationship with both the spinal cord and cerebellum but, as noted above, have very limited direct contact with the end organ.

The medial vestibular nucleus (MVN) lies just below the floor of the fourth ventricle medial to the LVN and inferior vestibular nucleus (IVN). Many primary afferents terminate in its rostral portion, mainly from the semicircular canals. Primary afferents from the saccule and utricle tend to terminate caudally, along the border shared with the IVN. MVN neurons from this same border region project axons to the ipsilateral flocculus, nodulus and uvula of the cerebellum. Commissural fibers enter the MVN from the contralateral SVN, MVN and IVN.

The inferior vestibular nucleus (IVN) is the most caudally located of the four major vestibular nuclei. This nucleus receives the greatest number of primary afferents, mainly from the saccule and utricle. The greatest representation is from the saccule and the least from the semicircular canals. Commissural fibers to the IVN arise from the contralateral MVN, SVN and IVN. It receives fibers from the ipsilateral SVN, and has reciprocal connections with the ipsilateral flocculonodular lobe.

EFFERENT FIBERS

A group of efferent fibers from the CNS course peripherally in the eighth nerve. They terminate on the cell bodies of Type II hair cells and on the afferent calyx associated with Type I hair cells. They originate bilaterally from small multipolar neurons located just lateral to the abducens nucleus and ventral to the MVN.[14] Duschesne and Sans suggested that efferent fibers that terminate on Type II cells are excitatory whereas efferents to the Type I hair cells are inhibitory.[16]

VESTIBULOSPINAL TRACTS

Lateral Vestibulospinal Tract

The lateral vestibulospinal tract (LVST) originates from cells located in the LVN[17] and from a much smaller number of cells in the IVN.[18] This tract descends ipsilaterally, contains rapidly conducting fibers and shifts from a ventrolateral position at cervical levels to a gradually more ventromedial position at lower levels (Figure 8). The LVST extends to all spinal cord levels, and terminals are found mainly in Rexed's laminae VII and VIII. Since motoneurons are found in lamina IX, the monosynaptic connections described below are probably on motoneuron dendrites that extend out of lamina IX. Neurons of the LVN project in a somatotopic pattern to all levels of the spinal cord. This pattern is reflected in the fact that cells located in the dorsocaudal LVN tend to project to lumbosacral levels, whereas cells located in the ventrorostral LVN tend to project to cervical levels.[19-21] This pattern, however, is complicated by the fact that collaterals of many LVST axons terminate at levels rostral to that of their final axon termination. Abzug and associates[22] showed that fifty percent of units tested at the cervical level also had axon terminals at upper lumbar levels. This indicates that at least two populations of LVST axons project to the cervical level. One population consists of terminal projections and the second, seen in Abzug and associates' study, consists of axon collaterals of fibers continuing on to lower levels. This second anatomical pattern also means that the cervical cord receives much of the same neurophysiological information that is sent to lumbosacral levels, suggesting coordination between fore- and hindlimb muscles.[23]

Stimulation of cells within the LVN results in excitatory postsynaptic

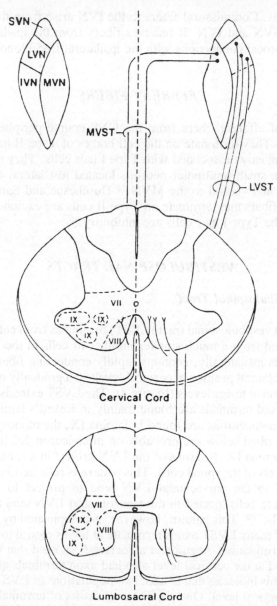

FIGURE 8. This is a schematic diagram of major vestibulospinal projections. The lateral vestibulo-spinal tract (LVST) terminates ipsilaterally in laminae VII and VIII at all levels. The medial vestibu-lospinal tract (MVST) descends in the medial longitudinal fasciculus only to upper thoracic levels. MVST axons project bilaterally to laminae VII and VIII. Superior vestibular nucleus, SVN; lateral vestibular nucleus, LVN; medial vestibular nucleus, MVN; inferior vestibular nucleus, IVN.

potentials (EPSP's) in ipsilateral dorsal neck and back muscle motoneurons. In many of these motoneurons the latencies were short enough to conclude that activation was monosynaptic.[21,24] Ipsilateral limb extensor motoneurons also respond with EPSP's when LVN neurons are stimulated. In some, the synaptic delay is short enough to assume monosynaptic connections. Cat hindlimb motoneurons that respond monosynaptically correspond with the quadriceps and gastrocnemius-soleus muscles. More typically, however, these and other hindlimb and forelimb motoneurons respond with di- or polysynaptic excitation.[21,25] Limb flexor motoneurons respond with an inhibitory postsynaptic potential (IPSP). These are disynaptic connections and involve an inhibitory interneuron located in the spinal cord gray.[25,26] In general, the LVST facilitates ipsilateral extensor musculature by way of spinal cord interneurons.

The ventrally located LVN neurons are the direct target of some primary vestibular afferents, implying that cervical motoneurons are under more direct vestibular control than are lumbosacral motoneurons.[27-29] The ventral LVN neurons also receive polysynaptic input, however, polysynaptic input is more widespread throughout the remainder of the LVN neurons.

Head tilt (side down) exciting the otolith receptors, facilitates activity in ipsilateral LVN neurons and in LVST axons.[30] Semicircular canal stimulation also has been reported to excite LVST neurons.[31]

In addition to reacting to labyrinthine input, LVST neurons also may be excited by direct electrical stimulation of limb and neck afferent nerves. The latency can be prolonged, especially from hindlimb nerves. The anatomical route is believed to include spinovestibular fibers[32] and collaterals of spinocerebellar fibers.[33] The facilitation is not powerful, but does influence a large number of both cervical and lumbosacral neurons, demonstrating an interaction of somatic and vestibular sensory inputs. The exact pattern of somatosensory facilitation of LVST neurons is dependent upon the presence or absence of the cerebellum.

The cerebellum has important connections with LVN neurons. These neurons are directly influenced by signals from fastigial nucleus cells and from Purkinje cells of the anterior and posterior vermis and paravermal cortex. Fastigial cells facilitate LVN neurons while Purkinje cells have an inhibitory effect. The excitatory effect via fastigial axons is widespread throughout the LVN showing no somatotopic organization[34] and may function to help maintain tonic activity of LVST neurons.[35] The flocculonodular lobe projects to the LVN, although more sparsely than to the other vestibular nuclei.[36] Stimulation of the flocculus, which would presumably excite the inhibitory Purkinje cells, does not produce IPSP's in LVST neurons. Nodulus Purkinje cells, however, can inhibit LVN neurons projecting back to the cerebellum, but effects on LVST neurons are lacking.[37] Anterior lobe Purkinje cell inhibition of LVST neurons has been reported and may be in response to stimulation of somatic afferent nerves.[38] In general, cerebellar cortical influence is greater in more dorsal portions of the LVN suggesting more intimate cerebellar involvement in hindlimb muscle activity.

In summary, the LVST follows a somatotopic organization with neurons projecting to the cervical spinal cord located ventrorostrally and lumbosacral neurons located dorsocaudally in the LVN. Primary afferent vestibular fibers that project to the LVN are found in ventral (cervical) portions and represent primarily the otolith organ but also the semicircular canals. Cerebellar input to the LVN tends to be more concentrated in dorsal (lumbosacral) portions. Stimulation of spinal nerves can excite LVST neurons and similar nerve stimulation also activates the cerebellar input. Stimulation of LVST neurons facilitates ipsilateral dorsal neck and axial muscles and ipsilateral limb extensor muscles.

Medial Vestibulospinal Tract

The medial vestibulospinal tract (MVST) originates from neurons located in the medial, inferior and lateral vestibular nuclei. The majority of MVST neurons lie in the rostral third of the MVN which receives primary canal and otolith afferents.[17,29,39] The remaining neurons are located in the border areas of the adjoining MVN, LVN and IVN.[18,40,41]

The axons of the MVST enter the medial longitudinal fasciculus (MLF) of both sides and descend into the spinal cord, to terminate in laminae VII and VIII. The distribution of the MVST differs somewhat from that of the LVST. The MVST terminates bilaterally, with fibers crossing in the brain stem, whereas the LVST is exclusively ipsilateral. The LVST terminates at all levels; however, the MVST extends caudally only to upper thoracic levels.[18]

Unlike the LVST, the MVST contains inhibitory as well as excitatory fibers.[24] Neurophysiological evidence shows that some inhibitory and excitatory fibers end monosynaptically on dorsal neck muscle motoneurons. Only excitatory fibers have been reported terminating on forelimb motoneurons. The inhibitory projections are both ipsilateral and contralateral with some bilateral projections to lower cervical segments.[25] Excitatory MVST fibers terminate contralaterally and bilaterally at lower cervical levels. Inhibition conveyed by the MVST may be restricted to axial musculature as no monosynaptic IPSP's have been reported for limb motoneurons.[21]

A large number of vestibular nucleus neurons which give rise to the MVST can be fired monosynaptically by stimulation of the ipsilateral vestibular nerve.[42] The proportion of these second-order neurons is greater in the MVST than in the LVST, implying that the rostral spinal cord, via the MVST, is under more direct vestibular control. Primary projections largely from the semicircular canals terminate in areas of the vestibular nuclear complex that give rise to the MVST.[43,44] Neck motoneurons can be excited disynaptically by stimulation of semicircular canal afferents;[45] however, MVST neurons also respond to otolith stimulation.[46] The anterior cerebellum provides inhibitory input to MVST neurons,[27] whereas input from the fastigial nucleus produces EPSP's.[47]

In summary, the MVST arises primarily from the rostral one third of the MVN which in turn, receives primary afferents, largely from the semicircular canals. The cerebellum also projects to cells of origin of the MVST. The MVST contains fibers that are both excitatory and inhibitory and projects caudally in the MLF on both sides as far as upper thoracic levels. Activity in the MVST appears to be concerned with adjustments in neck musculature to help maintain head stability in space. To this degree it aids in maintaining a stable platform in which the visual system operates.

RETICULOSPINAL TRACTS

Four nuclei located in the pontomedullary brain stem are responsible for the fibers of the reticulospinal tracts. These nuclei are the nucleus reticularis (NR) pontis oralis, NR pontis caudalis, NR gigantocellularis and NR ventralis. These nuclei give rise to the medial reticulospinal tract (MRST) and the lateral reticulospinal tract (LRST).

Lateral Reticulospinal Tract

The LRST arises medially from NR gigantocellularis and NR ventralis[48-50] and, therefore, is of medullary origin. Fibers descend in the ventrolateral funiculus ispsilaterally to all spinal cord levels, with some fibers descending on the contralateral side. Fibers terminate throughout the ventral horn and in the base of the dorsal horn.[39,51]

Medial Reticulospinal Tract

The MRST arises rostrally from NR pontis oralis, NR pontis caudalis and from the dorsal part of NR gigantocellularis[48-50] and, therefore, is primarily of pontine origin. It descends in the ventromedial funiculus to all spinal cord levels ipsilaterally with many of the axons extending to and beyond lumbar levels. It has some contralateral descending projections. Many long axons also give off collaterals at higher levels.[49] Most terminal endings are found throughout the ventral horn and, unlike the LRST, many fibers cross in the anterior commissure of the spinal cord. Both reticulospinal tracts contain many long axons with collaterals terminating at cervical levels. Termination of both tracts is primarily within lamina VII and VIII.

Vestibular and Cerebellar Projections to Reticular Nuclei

Both otolith and semicircular canal stimulation produces bilateral activation of reticular neurons; however this activation is indirect since monosynaptic excitation has not been reported.[10,52,53] Inhibition of the reticular neurons following labyrinthine stimulation is produced only polysynaptically.[54,55] LRST neurons appear to be more closely linked with vestibular input than are MRST neurons as measured by whole nerve stimulation;[55] however, the MRST neurons are more sensitive to isolated canal stimulation suggesting the MRST is more canal related.

Vestibular nuclear projections to the reticular formation are quite extensive and all four vestibular nuclei project to the reticular nuclei. Most of the vestibular signals reaching the reticular formation are higher order suggesting that signals from other sources are mixed with the vestibular signals.[54,56]

The cerebellum also projects to the reticular nuclei and appears to play a major role in shaping the output of the reticulospinal neurons. Cerebellectomy results in a marked reduction in the number of reticular neurons responding during locomotion and static tilt. Fastigial nucleus fibers terminate contralaterally throughout the medial pontomedullary reticular formation, reflecting fastigial influence on both the MVST and LRST. Information relayed by the fastigial nucleus is most likely from somatic or vestibular receptors. The dentate nucleus of the cerebellum projects to the ipsilateral pontine reticular formation[57] providing a close relationship with cerebral cortical motor systems.[58] The distribution of the dentatoreticular terminals suggests interaction with the MRST. Somatosensory input into the reticular formation has been recorded and is, in general, excitatory.[59-61] This input is from deep receptors but not from muscle spindle or Golgi tendon organs.[62,63] Reticular neurons show rapid habituation to continued somatic stimulation.[63]

Reticulospinal tract axon activity onto spinal cord interneurons shows these indirect pathways to be of importance in relaying vestibular and somatosensory influences.[64,65] Activation of fibers of the MRST excites both axial and limb muscle motoneurons including both flexor and extensor groups.[66-68] In comparison, the excitatory activity of the LRST axons is restricted to neck and back muscle motoneurons and these excitation effects seem to be more directed to specific muscle groups.

DESCENDING VESTIBULAR INFLUENCES

Vestibular signals interact in a complex manner with other systems to produce a number of postural reflexes. The cerebellum appears to play a key role in these interactions which can involve limb and neck proprioception, touch, vision and descending cortical influences relayed to the vestibular complex primarily via the reticular formation. The various sensory modalities interact to provide information to the posture control system from three frames of reference. These are: (1) proprioception, the sense of position and movement of one part of the body relative to another, via muscle, joint, tactile and visual receptors; (2) exteroception, the relationship of objects in the environment to each other, via primarily visual and tactile inputs; and (3) exproprioception, or information about the body parts relative to the external environment, from all types of sensory receptors. Because the vestibular system subserves a purely exproprioceptive sense that reports velocity and acceleration of the head relative to gravity and inertia, it is especially useful in correcting erroneous information from other sensory inputs.[69]

The vestibulospinal tracts carry more than just vestibular information and provide only one route by which postural reflexes are evoked. Disynaptic activation of extensor muscles directly from the labyrinth is possible; however, this direct route is probably not sufficient for the execution of most of the vestibular reflexes, which can be relatively complex depending upon the amplitude and frequency of the stimulus. Polysynaptic pathways involving both vestibulospinal and reticulospinal tracts are probably more important in producing the appropriate response.

Behavioral studies with patients who have little or no vestibular function has shown that an interesting sensory interrelationship exists between otolith input and input from other sensory systems used for balance control. As expected, these patients lose balance more easily than do normal subjects. A major cause for loss of balance is their failure to ignore false proprioceptive or visual signals. Apparently in normal subjects, visual and proprioceptive cues are constantly compared against the steady, static reference from the otolith system and are largely ignored if they do not match. In vestibular defective subjects, the otolith reference signal is missing.

The frequency response range of primary afferents from the otolith end organ extends up to at least 2.0 Hz;[9] however, within the CNS the otolith system threshold levels indicate that it is responsive only in the static or near static condition.[70] The slow dynamics of the system led Nashner[71] to conclude that the otolith system probably plays no role in the detection of body sway. Body sway represents a relatively dynamic condition and may be in the realm of semicircular canal function. Using cats with plugged semicircular canals, Schor[72] concluded that the otoliths are responsible for compensatory reflexes involving limb and neck muscles only at frequencies below 0.1 Hz. Responses above that frequency appear to result from semicircular canal excitation. Perhaps the CNS regulates the useable response range of the otolith organ.

If humans are dropped from 2.5 to 20.3 cm above the ground while in a standing position, EMG activity in both gastrocnemius and tibialis anterior muscles begins about 75 ms after the onset of the fall regardless of the fall height.[73] This is probably a long latency, otolith-initiated, pre-programmed control of landing, involving both extensor and flexor muscles. The complexity of the response suggests that the reflex incorporates vestibuloreticulospinal pathways as well as vestibulospinal pathways.

If cats are dropped from 40 to 50 cm above the ground, their muscles respond with EMG activity at 55 ms and again at about 70 to 100 ms. The early peak does not habituate with subsequent drops and its amplitude is a function of the amplitude of linear acceleration. If labyrinthectomized, the early response is lost, but the later response remains. If only the canals are removed, both responses remain intact.[74] These results indicate that the otoliths are responsible for the early response. Further studies showed that the latency of onset of the second EMG response is a function of fall height, and is dependent upon visual, tactile and proprioceptive cues. This second response probably represents a preprogrammed response in anticipation of landing and combines cues from several sensory sources.

Similar experiments performed on monkeys[75] and labyrinthine defective humans[76-78] produced similar results. The early EMG response is reduced in labyrinthine defective patients and abolished by labyrinthectomy in monkeys. The second EMG peak occurs at about the time of contact regardless of fall height. Lacour and associates[79] concluded that the early response may involve direct vestibulospinal pathways. Since responses involved flexor muscles they suggested that rapid vestibuloreticulospinal routes may also contribute.

VESTIBULO-OCULAR REFLEX

The vestibulo-ocular reflex (VOR) functions to help maintain a stable retinal image during head movements. In the primate this appears to be primarily a function of the semicircular canal system. The generation and control of eye movements by canal input is a complex task that uses both direct and indirect pathways between the vestibular nuclei and the oculomotor neuron nuclei (III, IV and VI). In addition, since the visual system also plays a role in stabilizing retinal images, interaction exists within the CNS between the vestibular and visual systems.

The VOR functions to support the visual system in its efforts to maintain a stable retinal image during head movements. When the head is motionless and the eyes are not moving in the head, the image from a stationary visual environment will remain stable on the retina. When the head is moved the retinal image will slide across the retina if the eyes remain fixed in their orbits. This may blur the image, depending upon the velocity of the head movement, but it would certainly cause the target on the fovea to slide off out of that narrow beam of "best vision". In addition, movement perceived by the peripheral retina would falsely signal that the environment was turning around us, and would probably lead to a loss of balance. The semicircular canals, and to a much lesser extent, the otoliths, detect head movements and through the VOR, reflexly move the eyes in the orbit at the same velocity as the head, but in the opposite direction, in order to compensate for the head movement. Perhaps the value of this system can be better appreciated by reading the account of a physician who describes the effects of his loss of vestibular function.[80]

The semicircular canals of humans are largely responsible for the control of vestibular reflex eye movements. Otolith stimulation can regulate eye position, but its effect in the human is slight.[81] Measuring the rate at which we can oscillate our heads, 7 Hz appears to be an approximate maximum frequency for natural head rotations.[82] Experimental studies have shown that the VOR responds with minimal distortion over the range of about 0.01-7 Hz.[83,84] The match of this frequency range underscores the relationship between the canals and the VOR.

The extraocular muscles are innervated by three cranial nerves: oculomotor (III), trochlear (IV), and abducens (VI). The abducens nucleus is located in the caudal pons, close to the rostral extent of the SVN. Abducens nerve fibers innervate the ipsilateral lateral rectus muscle which moves the eye laterally (abduction). The trochlear nucleus is found in the caudal mesencephalon. Its fibers cross as they exit the brainstem and terminate in the superior oblique muscle. The oculomotor nuclear complex is in the rostral mesencephalon and gives rise to fibers that innervate the remaining extraocular muscles, including the medial rectus which moves the eye medially (adduction). The oculomotor nucleus is subdivided according to the various muscles it innervates.[85-87]

The SVN and rostral MVN give rise to neurons that ascend in the brainstem to terminate in various oculomotor nuclei. Fibers from the SVN ascend in the ipsilateral medial longitudinal fasciculus (MLF) to terminate in the ipsilateral trochlear and in the oculomotor nuclei of both sides. Fibers from the MVN enter the abducens nuclei on both sides. Other MVN fibers enter the contralateral MLF and terminate in a pattern similar to that of the SVN. A second, less well known pathway, the ascending tract of Deiters', passes from the LVN to the oculomotor nucleus.[88]

The oculomotor plant includes the eye, its passive supportive tissues, muscles and motoneurons. When eye movements take place, the firing pattern of the motoneurons must be controlled to account for inertia of the eye, viscoelastic properties of the supportive tissues, as well as the desired displacement and velocity of the eye movement. A number of premotor neurons are located throughout the brainstem that provide the appropriate signals to drive the oculomotor motoneurons. These include burst, tonic, burst-tonic and pause cells, and seem to be concentrated in the paramedian pontine reticular formation (PPRF) for control of horizontal eye movements.[89-91]

The vestibulo-ocular reflex is, at its simplest, a three neuron reflex.[92] The three neuron reflex is made up of one neuron cell body in the eighth nerve, a second in the vestibular nuclear complex, and the third in one of the oculomotor nuclei. In order to move the eye to a new position, the extraocular muscles require a neurophysiological signal representing both head angular displacement and head angular velocity. The angular acceleration signal to the canal has been integrated once by the mechanics of the canal to provide an angular velocity signal. This signal must be mathematically integrated once again to provide the required angular displacement signal. This second integration is believed to take place within the CNS, probably involving the cerebellum and reticular formation.[84] In addition, the VOR interacts closely with visual feedback signals within the CNS. The three neuron reflex, therefore, is a critical part of the VOR, but is not enough by itself to accurately explain the operation of the VOR.

The rate of decay of the slow phase of postrotatory nystagmus was originally thought to be a direct reflection of the return of the cupula to its resting position.[11] The rate of decay of slow phase nystagmus was measured and from it the time constant of cupular return was calculated. The cupular time constant (T_c) is rate of return of the cupula to its resting position and, in this case, was measured as the rate of decay of slow phase postrotatory nystagmus. Another way to describe the time constant is to say that it is the time required for the cupula to return to 37% of its original position. In this original study T_c was estimated to be about 10 seconds.[11] This would mean that in 10 seconds the cupula had returned to 37% of its original position. In 20 seconds it had returned to 13.7% (.37 × .37) of its original position and in 30 seconds was almost completely at rest with only 5.1% deflection remaining (0.37 × 0.37 × 0.37). The response, however, was found to be affected by vision. With vision, nystagmus usually stops in less than a minute. In absolute darkness, the slow phase velocity decays, stops, then resumes again, but in the opposite direction often continuing for several minutes. Revised models of the VOR incorporate the reversed, or after nystagmus, and add an adaption time constant (T_a) to account for it.[93] Slow phase nystagmus recorded in absolute darkness, using this revised model, determined T_c to be 21s and T_a to be 80s.

Neurophysiological studies have shown that the T_c measured by slow phase nystagmus is not the same as T_c measured by activity in the peripheral afferent neurons. Using neurophysiological techniques, T_c in the cat is about 4s as compared with a nystagmus measurement of canal function

(T_{vor}) of 12s.[94] Fernandez and Goldberg[9] found a similar three-fold difference in peripheral nerve activity ($T_c = 5.7s$) as compared with eye movements ($T_{vor} = 16s$) in the monkey. Time constants can serve as quantitative estimates of VOR function and are more meaningful than measures of nystagmus duration since, theoretically, they represent actual nervous system substrates. The neuroanatomical substrates of the various time constants, however, are not yet conclusively established.

The transformation of T_c to T_{vor} takes place in the vestibular nuclei. This transformation enables the VOR to operate accurately at lower frequencies of head movement. In the vestibular nuclei, a second signal is added to T_c and, since this second signal disappears with anesthesia, it is presumed to be coming from other CNS structures,[95] and may represent information from the optokinetic system.[84] The T_{vor} signal is proportional to head velocity. In order to be effective in producing the desired eye movement, the oculomotor motoneuron must receive both an eye velocity and an eye position signal. The conversion of the eye velocity signal to an eye position signal does not take place in the vestibular nuclei, but probably involves neurons in the cerebellum, brainstem reticular formation, or both.[84]

Another measure of the VOR, gain, may be a more direct measure of the effectiveness of canal stimulation in maintaining a stable image on the retina. Gain is the ratio of head angular motion to eye angular motion. When the head is turned, if the eyes compensate by turning exactly the same degree but in the opposite direction, the gain is 1.0, and the retinal image remains stationary. (Actually the gain is -1.0 because of the opposite direction of the eye movements, but we will ignore the minus sign for now.) If the eyes turn less than the head, gain is less than 1.0. Since this eye movement response represents the purpose of the VOR, gain is logically the most meaningful measure of VOR performance. When tested in the dark, with a subject alert and performing mental arithmetic, gain is about 0.65.[96] If the subject becomes drowsy, gain becomes much less and nystagmus will habituate.[97] If the subject is asked to look at an imaginary spot on the wall, however, gain rises to about 0.95.[95] Arousal also interacts significantly with other measures involving slow phase eye movements, such as the time constants and nystagmus duration.

In considering only the horizontal VOR, signals arrive in the rostral MVN from the semicircular canal proportional to head velocity with a cupular time constant (T_c). The exact excitatory pathways to the eye muscle motoneurons are not fully understood, and the following is somewhat speculative. In the vestibular nuclei a signal, probably from the optokinetic system, is added to increase the value of T_c to the value of T_{vor} (about 20s). Second order fibers leave the MVN, cross the midline and terminate in the contralateral abducens nucleus (Figure 9). Other second order fibers, not shown in Figure 9, ascend in the ipsilateral MLF directly

Compensatory
eye movements

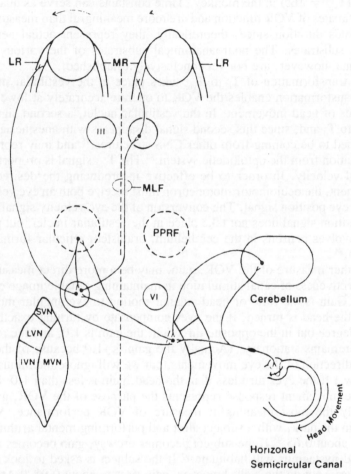

FIGURE 9. Major excitatory connections of the horizontal vestiblo-ocular reflex are shown diagrammatically. Primary afferents project to the vestibular nuclei and cerebellum. Secondary fibers project to the abducens nucleus (VI) and to the paramedian pontine reticular formation (PPRF). Ascending internuclear fibers in the medial longitudinal fasciculus (MLF) terminate in the oculomotor nuclear complex (III). Contraction of appropriate medial rectus (MR) and lateral rectus (LR) extraocular muscles produce compensatory eye movements in the direction opposite to that of the head movement.

to the oculomotor nuclear complex. Eye position commands, probably from the PPRF, are added at the MVN and at the abducens nucleus. The abducens nucleus send fibers to the lateral rectus muscle to abduct the eye on the same side. Internuclear neurons within the abducens nucleus give rise to axons that cross the midline and ascend in the MLF to the contra-lateral medial rectus subnucleus of the oculomotor nuclear complex. The ascending internuclear fibers in the MLF, therefore, carry a completely assembled motoneuron signal. Oculomotor nucleus motoneurons project to the medial rectus muscle on that side to adduct the eye.

In addition to the processing described above, additional signals are coordinated at the motoneuron. Saccades move the eye in the direction opposite to the slow phase movement, so the slow phase signal must be in-hibited and a burst of activity added to contract the antagonistic muscle. These other influences are believed to originate in cells located in the pon-tine or mesencephalic reticular formation[98,99] with similar influences af-fecting vertical eye movements originating from structures located more rostrally.

SUMMARY

The vestibular end organ is made up of mechanical transducers special-ized to detect linear and angular acceleration over the range of physiolog-ical head movements. The semicircular canals are specialized to respond to dynamic head movements whereas the otoliths appear to function predominantly in the static sphere. The neuroepithelium of the utricle and saccule, and semicircular canals have many structures in common, including reception of efferent fibers which provide a pathway by which the CNS can regulate or balance input signals to the CNS from the ear.

Descending pathways responsible for postural reflexes include the ves-tibulospinal and reticulospinal tracts. Both receive signals from the vestib-ular end organ and both are strongly influenced by cerebellar efferents. Descending control of neck musculature is more closely linked to the vestibular end organ and to the semicircular canals. Limb muscle reflexes are more closely linked to input from several sensory systems. The MVST is strongly influenced by semicircular canal signals and reflexly controls neck musculature. The LVST is involved with control of both neck and limb muscles and has close links with the cerebellum. The reticulospinal tracts are also involved in postural reflexes and appear to be influenced by vestibular as well as other sensory stimuli.

Otolith input may be of primary importance as a stable gravity sensitive reference signal against which other balance cues are compared. More dynamic movements associated with body sway may be handled by the semicircular canal system.

The VOR aids in body equilibrium during head movements by pro-viding stability of the eyeball with reference to the visual environment. The signal from the vestibular end organ, primarily the semicircular canals, is modified at successive levels of the VOR to provide a signal appropriate for the eye muscle motoneurons. Some modifications occur at the vestibular nuclear complex and represent feedback from the visual system as well as input from the cerebellum and from the reticular formation.

The vestibular system is a complex sensory and motor system capable of influencing tone in a large number of body muscles. All evidence indicates that a primary function of the system is to help maintain spatial orientation and body equilibrium. Descending vestibular influences regulate postural muscles in a relatively direct fashion; however, a neuroanatomical analysis reveals that the vestibulospinal system can accomplish its goal only with the close cooperation of the cerebellum and reticular system to name only two of the better known cooperating systems. Since, in the human, vision is an especially important source of equilibrium cues, ascending vestibular influences support spatial orientation primarily through interaction with the oculomotor and visual systems.

A quantitative approach to vestibular reflexes, and especially the VOR, promises to provide knowledge of the specific anatomical site of each component of the various related reflexes. Localization of the anatomical substrates of the VOR will help us to identify the site of the contributing abnormality in populations with non-normal nystagmus. Knowledge of the details of the complex interaction of vestibular and nonvestibular pathways provides the potential for more accurate hypotheses to account for the reported beneficial therapeutic effects of vestibular system stimulation. With an expanded understanding of the structure and function of the vestibular system, coupled with continued awareness of basic and clinical research results, the therapist will be better equipped to use this system for both diagnosis and therapy on a day-to-day basis.

REFERENCES

1. Anson BJ, Bast TH: The ear and temporal bone: Development and adult structure, in Coats GM, Schench HP, Miller HV (eds): *Otolaryngology.* Hagerstown, MD, Prior, 1955.

2. Hardy M: Observations on the innervations of the macula sacculi in man. *Anat Rec* 59:403-418, 1934.

3. Ades, HW, Engstrom H: Form and innervation of the vestibular epithelia, in *The Role of the Vestibular Organs in the Exploration of Space.* NASA SP-77, 1965, p 30.

4. Wersall J, Lundquist PG: Morphological polarization of the mechano-receptors of the vestibular and acoustic systems, in *Second Symposium on the Role of the Vestibular Organs in Space Exploration.* NASA SP-115, 1966, pp 57-72.

5. Lowenstein O, Sand A: The individual and integrated activity of the semi-circular canals of the elasmobranch labyrinth. *J Physiol* 99: 89-101, 1940.

6. Lowenstein O: The effect of galvanic polarization on the impulse discharge from sense endings in the isolated labyrinth of the thornback ray (Raja Clavata). *J Physiol* 127: 104-117, 1955.

7. Spoendlin HH: Discussion of: The functional significance of the ultra-structure of the vestibular end organs, in *Second Symposium on the Role of the Vestibular Organs in Space Exploration.* NASA SP-115, 1966, p 89.

8. Spoendlin HH: Ultrastructural studies of the labyrinth in squirrel monkey, in *The Role of the Vestibular Organs in the Exploration of Space.* NASA SP-77, 1965, pp 7-22.

9. Fernandez C, Goldberg JM: Physiology of peripheral neurons innervating otolith organs of the squirrel monkey. III. Response dynamics. *J Neurophysiol* 39:996-1008, 1976.

10. Goldberg JM, Fernandez C: Responses of peripheral vestibular neurons to angular and linear accelerations in the squirrel monkey. *Acta Otolaryngol* 80:101-110, 1975.

11. vonEgmond AAJ, Groen JJ, Jongkees LBW: The mechanism of the semicircular canal. *J Physiol* 110:1-17, 1949.

12. Robinson D: The mechanics of the human saccadic eye movement. *J Physiol* 174:245, 1964.

13. Abend WK: Functional organization of the superior vestibular nucleus of the squirrel monkey. *Brain Res* 132:65-84, 1977.

14. Gacek RR: Afferent and efferent innervation of the labyrinth. *Adv Oto-Rhino-Laryngol* 28: 1-13, 1982.

15. Carleton SC, Carpenter MB: Afferent and efferent connections of the medial, inferior and lateral vestibular nuclei in the cat and monkey. *Brain Res* 278:29-51, 1983.

16. Duschesne C, Sans A: Control of the vestibular nerve activity by the efferent system in the cat. *Acta Otolaryngol* 90:82-85, 1980.

17. Brodal A, Pompeiano O, Walberg F: *The Vestibular Nuclei and their Connections.* London, Oliver and Boyd, 1962.

18. Rapoport S, Susswein A, Uchino Y, Wilson VJ: Properties of vestibular neurones projecting to neck segments of the cat spinal cord. *J Physiol* 268:493-510, 1977.

19. Peterson BW: Distribution of neural responses to tilting within vestibular nuclei of the cat. *J Neurophysiol* 33:750-767, 1970.

20. Pompeiano O, Brodal A: Spino-vestibular fibers in the cat. An experimental study. *J Comp Neurol* 108:353-382, 1957.

21. Wilson VJ, Yoshida M: Comparison of effects of stimulation of Deiters' nucleus and medial longitudinal fasciculus on neck, forelimb and hindlimb motoneurons. *J Neurophysiol* 32:742-758, 1969.

22. Abzug, C, Maeda M, Peterson BW, Wilson VJ: Cervical branching of lumbar vestibulospinal axons. *J Physiol* 243:499-522, 1974.

23. Chan CWY: Tonic labyrinthine reflex control of limb posture: Re-examination of the classical concept. *Adv Neurol* 39:621-632, 1983.

24. Akaike T, Fanardjian VV, Ito M, Ohno T: Electrophysiological analysis of the vestibulospinal reflex pathway of rabbit. II. Synaptic actions upon spinal neurons. *Exp Brain Res* 17:497-515, 1973.

25. Grillner S, Hongo T, Lund S: The vestibulospinal tract: Effects on alpha motoneurons in the lumbosacral spinal cord in the cat. *Exp Brain Res* 10:94-120, 1970.

26. Hultborn M, Illert M, Santini M: Convergence on interneurons mediating the reciprocal Ia inhibition of motoneurons. III. Effects from supra-spinal pathways. *Acta Physiol Scand* 96:368-391, 1976.

27. Akaike T, Fanardjian VV, Ito M, Nakajima H: Cerebellar control of vestibulospinal tract cells in rabbit. *Exp Brain Res* 18:446-463, 1973.

28. Ito M, Hongo T, Okado Y: Vestibular-evoked postsynaptic potentials in Deiters' neurons. *Exp Brain Res* 7:214-230, 1969.

29. Wilson VJ, Wylie RM, Marco LA: Projection to the spinal cord from the medial and descending vestibular nuclei of the cat. *Nature* 215:429-430, 1967.

30. Orlovsky GN, Parlova GA: Vestibular response of neurons of different descending pathways in cats with intact cerebellum and in decerebellated ones (in Russian). *Neirofizologiya* 4:303-310, 1972.

31. Fukushima K, Peterson BW, Wilson VJ: Vestibulospinal, reticulospinal and interstitiospinal pathways in the cat, in Granit R, Pompeiano O (eds): *Progress in Brain Research. Reflex Control of Posture and Movements.* Amsterdam, Elsevier, 50:121-136, 1979.

32. Pompeiano O, Brodal A: The origin of vestibulospinal fibers in the cat. An experimental-anatomical study, with comments on the descending medial longitudinal fasciculus. *Arch Ital Biol* 95:166-195, 1957.

33. Ito M, Kawai N, Udo M, Mano N: Axon reflex activation of Deiters' neurons from the cerebellar cortex through collaterals of the cerebellar afferents. *Exp Brain Res* 8:249-268, 1969.

34. Ito M, Udo M, Mano N, Kawai N: Synaptic action of the fastigiobulbar impulses upon neurons in the medullary reticular formation and vestibular nuclei. *Exp Brain Res* 11:29-47, 1970.

35. Wilson VJ, Peterson BW: Vestibulospinal and reticulospinal systems, in Brookhart JM,

Mountcastle VB (eds): *Handbook of Physiology: The Nervous System.* Bethesda, MD, Amer Physiol Soc, 2:667-702, 1981.

36. Brodal A, Pompeiano O, Walberg F: The anatomy of the vestibular nuclei and their connections, in Kornhuber HM (ed): *Handbook of Sensory Physiology. Vestibular System.* Berlin, Springer-Verlag, 6:239-352, 1974.

37. Precht W, Volkind R, Maeda M, Giretti ML: The effects of stimulating the cerebellar nodulus in the cat on the response of vestibular neurons. *Neuroscience* 1:301-312, 1976.

38. Bruggencate G, Scherer J, Teichmann R: Neuronal activity in the lateral vestibular nucleus of the cat. V. Topographical distribution of inhibitory effects mediated by the spino-olivocerebellar pathway. *Pfluegers Arch* 360:321-336, 1975.

39. Nyberg-Hansen R, Mascitti TA: Sites and mode of termination of fibers of the vestibulospinal tract in the cat. An experimental study with silver impregnation methods. *J Comp Neurol* 122: 369-388, 1964.

40. Akaike T: Comparison of neuronal composition of the vestibulospinal system between cat and rabbit. *Exp Brain Res* 18:429-432, 1973.

41. Akaike T, Fanardjian VV, Ito M et al.: Electrophysiological analysis of the vestibulospinal reflex pathway of rabbit. I. Classification of tract cells. *Exp Brain Res* 17:477, 1973.

42. Wilson VJ, Wylie RM, Marco LA: Synaptic inputs to cells in the medial vestibular nucleus. *J Neurophysiol* 31:176-185, 1968.

43. Precht W, Grippo J, Wagner A: Contribution of different types of central vestibular neurons to the vestibulospinal system. *Brain Res* 4:119-123, 1967.

44. Shimazu H, Precht W: Inhibition of central vestibular neurons from the contralateral labyrinth and its mediating pathway. *J Neurophysiol* 29:467-492, 1966.

45. Wilson VJ, Maeda M: Connections between semicircular canals and neck motoneurons in the cat. *J Neurophysiol* 37:346-357, 1974.

46. Goldberg JM, Fernandez C: Vestibular system, in Darian-Smith I (ed): *Handbook of Physiology. Sensory Processes.* Bethesda, MD, Amer Physiol Soc, 1984.

47. Shimazu M, Smith CM: Cerebellar and labyrinthine influences on single vestibular neurons identified by natural stimuli. *J Neurophysiol* 34:493-508, 1971.

48. Ito M, Udo M, Mano N: Long inhibitory and excitatory pathways converging onto cat reticular and Deiters' neurons and their relevance to reticulo-fugal axons. *J Neurophysiol* 33:210-266, 1970.

49. Peterson BW, Fillon M, Felpel LP, Abzug C: Responses of medial reticular neurons to stimulation of the vestibular nerve. *Exp Brain Res* 22:335-350, 1975.

50. Petras JM: Cortical, tectal and tegmental fiber connections in the spinal cord of the cat. *Brain Res* 6:275-324, 1967.

51. Nyberg-Hansen R: Sites and mode of termination of reticulo-spinal fibers in the cat. An experimental study with silver impregnation methods. *J Comp Neurol* 124:71-99, 1965.

52. Duensing F, Schaeffer KP: Die Aktivitat einzelmer Neurone der Formatio reticularis des nicht gefesselten Kaninchens bei Kopfwendungen und vestibularen Reizen. *Arch Psychiatr Nervenkr* 201:97-122, 1960.

53. Spyer KM, Ghelarducci B, Pompeiano O: Gravity responses of neurons in main reticular formation. *J Neurophysiol* 37:705-721, 1974.

54. Peterson BW, Abzug C: Properties of projections from vestibular nuclei to medial reticular formation in the cat. *J Neurophysiol* 38:1421-1435, 1975.

55. Peterson BW, Maunz RA, Pitts NG, Mackel R: Patterns of projection and branching of reticulospinal neurons. *Exp Brain Res* 23:333-351, 1975.

56. Ladpli R, Brodal A: Experimental studies of commissural and reticular formation projections from the vestibular nuclei in the cat. *Brain Res* 8:65-96, 1968.

57. Bantli M, Bloedel JR: Monosynaptic activation of a direct reticulospinal pathway by the dentate nucleus. *Pfluegers Arch* 357:236-242, 1975.

58. Thach WT: Timing of activity in cerebellar dentate nucleus and cerebral motor cortex during prompt volitional movement. *Brain Res* 88:233-241, 1975.

59. Eccles JC, Nicoll RA, Schwarz WF et al.: Reticulospinal neurons with and without monosynaptic inputs from cerebellar nuclei. *J Neurophysiol* 38:513-530, 1975.

60. Magni F, Willis WD: Subcortical and peripheral control of brain stem reticular neurons. *Arch Ital Biol* 102:434-448, 1964.

61. Peterson BW, Anderson ME, Filion M: Responses of pontomedullary reticular neurons to cortical, tectal, and cutaneous stimuli. *Exp Brain Res* 21:19-44, 1974.

62. Pompeiano O, Swett JE: Actions of graded cutaneous and muscle afferent volleys on brain stem units in the decerebrate, cerebellectomized cat. *Arch Ital Biol* 101:552-583, 1963.

63. Segundo JP, Takenada T, Encabo M: Somatic sensory properties of bulbar reticular neurons. *J Neurophysiol* 30:1221-1238, 1967.

64. Engberg I, Lundberg A, Ryall RW: Reticulospinal inhibition of transmission in reflex pathways. *J Physiol* 194:201-223, 1968.

65. Engberg I, Lundberg A, Ryall RW: Reticulospinal inhibition of interneurones. *J Physiol* 194:225-236, 1968.

66. Peterson BW: Reticulo-motor pathways: Their connections and possible roles in motor behavior, in Asanuma H, Wilson VJ (eds): *Integration in the Nervous System*. Tokyo, Igaku Shoin, 1979, pp 185-200.

67. Peterson BW, Pitts NG, Fukushima K: Reticulospinal connections with limb and axial motoneurons. *Exp Brain Res* 36:1-20, 1979.

68. Wilson VJ, Yoshida M, Schor RH: Supraspinal monosynaptic excitation and inhibition of thoracic back motoneurons. *Exp Brain Res* 11:282-295, 1970.

69. Nashner LM: Analysis of stance posture in humans, in Towle AL, Luschei ES (eds): *Handbook of Behavioral Neurobiology*, vol 5, *Motor Coordination*. New York, Plenum Press, 1981, pp 527-565.

70. Young LR, Meiry JL: A revised dynamic otolith model. *Aerospace Med* 39:606-608, 1968.

71. Nashner LM: A model describing the vestibular detection of body sway motion. *Acta Otolaryngol* 72:429-436, 1971.

72. Schor RH: Otolith contribution to neck and forelimb vestibulospinal reflexes. *Prog Oculomotor Res* 12:351-356, 1981.

73. Melville-Jones G, Watt DGD: Observations on the control of stepping and hopping movements in man. *J Physiol* 219:709-729, 1971.

74. Watt DGD: Responses of cats to sudden falls: An otolith originating reflex assisting landing. *J Physiol* 39:257-265, 1976.

75. Lacour M, Vidal PP, Xerri C: Early directional influence of visual motion cues on postural control in the falling monkey. *Ann NY Acad Sci* 374:403-411, 1981.

76. Greenwood RJ, Hopkins AP: Muscle activity in falling man. *J Physiol* 241:26-27P, 1974.

77. Greenwood RJ, Hopkins AP: Muscle responses during sudden falls in man. *J Physiol* 254:507-518, 1976.

78. Greenwood R, Hopkins AP: Motor control during stepping and falling in man, in Desmedt JE (ed): *Progress in Clinical Neurophysiology. Spinal and Supraspinal Mechanisms of Voluntary Motor Control*. Basel, Karger, 1980, pp 294-309.

79. Lacour M, Vidal PP, Xerri C: Dynamic characteristics of vestibular and visual control of rapid postural adjustments. *Adv Neurol* 39:589-606, 1983.

80. JC: Living without a balancing mechanism. *N Eng J Med* 246:458-460, 1952.

81. Miller EF: Counter-rolling of the human eyes produced by head tilt with respect to gravity. *Acta Otolaryngol* 54:479-501, 1962.

82. Skavenski AA, Hansen RM, Steinman RM, Winterson BJ: Quality of retinal image stabilization during small natural and artificial body rotations in man. *Vision Res* 19:675-683, 1979.

83. Landers PH, Taylor A: Transfer function analysis of the vestibulo-ocular reflex in the conscious cat, in Lennerstrand G, Bach-y-Rita P (eds): *Basic Mechanisms of Ocular Motility and Their Clinical Implications*. Oxford, Pergamon 24:505-508, 1975.

84. Robinson DA: Control of eye movements, in Brookhart JM, Mountcastle VB (eds): *Handbook of Physiology: The Nervous System*. Bethesda, MD, Amer Physiol Soc 2:1275-1320, 1981.

85. Warwick R: Representation of the extraocular muscles in the oculomotor nuclei of the monkey. *J Comp Neurol* 98:449-504, 1953.

86. Tarlov E, Tarlov SR: The representation of the extraocular muscles in the oculomotor nuclei: Experimental studies in the cat. *Brain Res* 34:35-52, 1971.

87. Gacek RR: Localization of neurons supplying the extraocular muscles in the kitten using horseradish peroxidase. *Exp Neurol* 44:381-403, 1974.

88. Gacek RR: Location of brain stem neurons projecting to the oculomotor nucleus in the cat. *Exp Neurol* 57:725-749, 1977.

89. Gouras P: Oculomotor system, in Kandel ER, Schwartz JH (eds): *Principles of Neural Science*. New York, Elsevier/North-Holland, 1981.

90. Galiana HL, Outerbridge JH: A bilateral model for central neural pathways in vestibulo-ocular reflex. *J Neurophysiol* 51:210-241, 1984.

91. Shimazu H: Neuronal organization of the premotor system controlling horizontal conjugate eye movements and vestibular nystagmus. *Adv Neurol* 39:565-588, 1983.

92. Szentagothi J: The elementary vestibulo-ocular reflex arc. *J Neurophysiol* 13:395-407, 1950.

93. Malcolm R, Melville-Jones G: A quantitative study of vestibular adaptation in humans. *Acta Otolaryngol* 70:126-135, 1970.

94. Melville-Jones G, Milsum JH: Frequency-response analysis of central vestibular unit activity resulting from rotational stimulation of the semicircular canals. *J Physiol* 219:191-215, 1971.

95. Buttner UW, Buttner U, Henn V: Transfer characteristics of neurons in vestibular nuclei of the alert monkey. *J Neurophysiol* 41:1614-1628, 1978.

96. Barr CC, Schultheis LW, Robinson DA: Voluntary non-visual control of the human vestibulo-ocular reflex. *Acta Otolaryngol* 81:365-375, 1976.

97. Collins WE: Effects of mental set upon vestibular nystagmus. *J Exp Psychol* 63:191-197, 1962.

98. Buttner V, Buttner-Ennever JA, Henn V: Vertical eye movement related unit activity in the rostral mesencephalic reticular formation of the alert monkey. *Brain Res* 130:239-252, 1977.

99. Keller EL: Participation of medial pontine reticular formation in eye movement generation in monkey. *J Neurophysiol* 37:316-332, 1974.

Assessment of Vestibular Function in Children

Patricia Montgomery, PhD, RPT

INTRODUCTION

The development of assessment techniques related to normal and abnormal functioning of the human vestibular system has lagged behind the development of methods to assess functioning of other sensory systems within the central nervous system. The relatively slow progress in understanding vestibular functions and in devising methods to test these functions is related to several factors. First, the minute size of the labyrinth and its relative inaccessibility for experimentation have made the peripheral end organ difficult to study. Second, as indicated in the preceding paper the neurophysiological connections between the vestibular nuclei in the brainstem and other central nervous system structures are vast in number and complexity, so that no single assessment technique can provide information on all the functions in which the vestibular system is known to play a role. Because of this second factor assessment of vestibular function has taken several divergent paths. Historically, the focus of vestibular assessment has been in two general areas: vestibular-ocular interactions and postural mechanisms. The purpose of this paper is to review these two major approaches to vestibular assessment (vestibular-ocular and postural) with emphasis on developmental applications.

VESTIBULAR-OCULAR TESTS

Neurophysiological Rationale

As the human subject surveys the visual environment, head and body movements pose a threat to the programming of accurate eye movements and to visual processing. The central nervous system, however, has developed an intimate relationship between the inner ear and cranial nerve nuclei governing eye movements. The "vestibular-ocular reflex"

Patricia Montgomery is a pediatric physical therapist involved in private practice and consultation with Therapeutic Intervention Programs, Inc. Address correspondence to 2217 Glenhurst Road, St. Louis Park, MN 55416.

or VOR is designed to maintain a stable retinal image when the head is moved. For example, movement of the head in one direction results in a compensatory eye movement in the opposite direction. The amount of literature (animal and human) describing vestibular-ocular pathways and the VOR is voluminous. Neural impulses from the labyrinth via the vestibular nuclei synapse in cranial nerve nuclei III (Oculomotor), IV (Trochlear), and VI (Abducens) as discussed in the previous paper. Three main vestibular-ocular pathways have been traced in animals, including routes through the medial longitudinal fasciculus, the brachium conjunctivium and the ascending tract of Deiters.[1] These pathways are long and, therefore, provide numerous opportunities to be influenced by other central nervous system mechanisms—both excitatory and inhibitory. This suggests that therapists should reject the notion that vestibular-ocular interaction is simple and that testing of nystagmus responses will provide comprehensive information regarding the functioning of the vestibular system (even of the vestibular-ocular mechanism). In addition, most methods to assess vestibular-ocular interaction involve eliciting some type of nystagmus (observed clinically as a rhythmic back and forth movement of the eyes, slow in one direction and fast in the opposite direction), rather than by studying the VOR in a natural situation.

Methodological Considerations

Types of Nystagmus. A spontaneous nystagmus (direction fixed and beating with similar intensity in all head positions) with the eyes closed is normally detected in a significant proportion of the normal population,[2] however, this type of nystagmus is strongly suppressed by visual fixation. When the eyes are open in light, a spontaneous nystagmus is almost always pathologic, although it is often the result of deficits in visual fixation reflexes, rather than the result of vestibular deficits. Congenital nystagmus (high frequency horizontal oscillations of the eyes during attempted fixation of stationary targets) is an ocular motor disorder which is the result of defective fixational reflexes.[3]

Positional nystagmus refers to nystagmus which occurs in certain head positions only and this information is useful as a diagnostic tool in determining central versus peripheral etiology.

Nystagmus can be elicited in a variety of manners. An optokinetic nystagmus (OKN) is elicited via a visual stimulus such as a rotating drum with black and white stripes. A filmstrip of cartoon characters or animals which is moved across the visual field can be used to elicit an OKN in children. Another approach is to study vestibular-visual interaction by rotating the individual while he is surrounded by a visual environment designed to elicit an OKN (i.e., white curtain with black design).

Thermal stimulation to the ear using air or water (caloric tests) will produce a nystagmus and is most helpful in determining unilateral deficits. Other methods test the vestibular apparatus bilaterally and may not be as useful in determining defects limited to one side.

Angular acceleration or deceleration is used to provide a more natural stimulus to the labyrinth. Electrically controlled or hand-operated rotating or oscillating chairs or turntables may be used. A torsion swing, or chair, which provides alternating angular accelerations of 180 degrees to the right and left at a rate of 10 revolutions per 60 seconds was recommended by the Eviatars for use with children.[4] Perrotatory nystagmus refers to eye movements occurring during movement, while postrotatory nystagmus refers to eye movements which occur following cessation of stimulation. Primary nystagmus is the nystagmus elicited immediately following a period of angular acceleration, either during constant velocity or after cessation of movement. Secondary nystagmus refers to a reversal in direction of eye movements which may occur following a primary nystagmus.

Parameters. As early as 1923, Holsopple stated that "one of the most characteristic features of all reported nystagmus measurements is the lack of uniformity of results among different investigators".[5(p285)] He identified three possible causes for these differences: (1) differences in the physiologic condition of the subjects, (2) differences in methods of applying stimuli, and (3) differences in methods of measuring results.

As research in vestibular assessment progressed, some of the variables which produced different test results were identified. Physiologic factors such as age, whether the individual is in an alert state, and the presence of certain drugs have been shown to alter the nystagmus response.[6,7] Such variables as whether the eyes are open or closed, whether testing is done in the dark or light, and the interval between tests will also affect the nystagmus response.

Several parameters are used to measure nystagmus. Before a more sophisticated method was developed for recording eye movements, nystagmus duration was the measure of choice and was usually timed with a stop-watch.[5] When more quantitative methods of measuring eye movements using the corneoretinal potential were developed, a wider range of nystagmus parameters could be measured. These include latency of response, frequency of beats, amplitude, and eye speed during the fast and slow phases of nystagmus.

Several issues related to vestibulo-ocular parameters should be considered by therapists. First, *duration* is considered by many authors to be a poor measure of vestibular sensitivity.[8-11] Henriksson investigated the relationship between speed of eye movement in the slow phase of perrotatory nystagmus and the vestibular stimulus during varying periods of constant velocity accelerations.[8] Subjects were tested in a darkened room in a revolving chair. The result was that eye-speed was approximately proportional (varied linearly) to a given stimulus (acceleration × time). The response was fairly constant for an individual subject, however, differences between subjects were large. In another test condition the subjects were accelerated to 66 degrees/second and, following 5 minutes of constant velocity, the chair was braked and stopped within 3 seconds. In this condition, the correlation between speed of eye movement and duration of nystagmus was poor.

In another study, Henriksson found that when identical caloric stimuli were used in adult subjects, duration seemed more constant than maximum eye speed.[11] With increasing stimuli, however, duration increased very little, while maximum eye speed more closely reflected the values of stimulation. For this reason he regarded nystagmus duration as an expression of "stiffness" in reaction rather than an expression of the excitatory effect of the stimulus on the sensory mechanism and recommended that eye speed be used as the expression of sensitivity of the vestibular apparatus in caloric tests.

The interaction of various nystagmus parameters during caloric and rotatory stimulations was also studied by Torok.[9] Clockwise and counterclockwise rotatory stimulations were applied to 17 adult subjects at an acceleration rate of 2.5 degrees/second^2 to constant velocities of 30, 45, 60, 90, and 180 degrees/second with a 5 minute interval between stimuli. Thirteen subjects received graded thermal (caloric) stimuli. Frequency of nystagmus beats and eye speed during the slow component were considered the best expressions of nystagmus intensity. Frequency is based on the fast component (due to interruption of the slow component), while maximum eye speed reflects the slow component. Torok suggested that frequency is the most relevant measure in caloric testing, while for lower rotatory accelerations, eye speed is the best measure and for stronger rotatory accelerations, frequency is the more consistent measure. Some authors, however, suggest that the great variability of the caloric nystagmus response among normal subjects makes insidious bilateral vestibular damage difficult to detect with this type of testing.[12]

Tibbling studied the nystagmus response of 84 children between 0 and 15 years of age to angular accelerations of 120 degrees/sec^2 for 1.8 seconds, followed by 1 minute of constant velocity.[10] Electronystagmography (ENG) recordings of perrotatory eye movements were made of the speed of the slow and fast components at 2,4,10,18 and 30 seconds following the start of rotation. The amplitudes at these points, frequency of beats per 10 seconds of rotation and the duration of the perrotatory nystagmus were also calculated. Tibbling stated that a high speed of the slow component is an expression of high peripheral activity of the vestibular system. She found that the youngest children had a very high maximum speed of the slow component, reflecting a vestibular response which was more intense than that of the older children in the study. Because she observed that a short duration nystagmus could be combined with a high maximum speed of the slow component, she concluded that duration is a poor parameter of the strength of vestibular reactivity in children. Since the amplitude of the response depends on when the slow phase is interrupted by the fast phase (considered to reflect central rather than vestibular activity), amplitude is considered to be a centrally evoked parameter. Tibbling concluded that nystagmus intensity could be classified according to peripheral activity (maximum speed of slow component) or central activity (amplitude).

In a study of full-term and premature infants using perrotatory nystagmus (torsion swing) and ice cold caloric (ICC), the number of beats per 10 seconds and the speed of the slow component were the most reliable measurements, whereas duration of nystagmus was much more variable.[13]

In summarizing parameters of nystagmus, McCabe stated that the maximum velocity of the slow component, measured in degrees per second, most closely correlates with cupular deflection and is the most frequently used index of the vestibular response.[14] Beat frequency over a ten-second period is also a measure of vestibular sensitivity, but is more variable and affected more by drugs, state of wakefulness and attentiveness. McCabe concluded that nystagmus duration is the least valuable parameter in vestibular testing.

Implications for the Clinician

Since the speed of eye movement in the slow phase of nystagmus has been suggested to be one of the most sensitive measures of vestibular function, this dictates the use of ENG. Nystagmus should also be elicited in light-proof rooms to exclude the potent variable of visual fixation. The use of sophisticated equipment would obviously result in more precise and reliable data regarding nystagmus parameters, however, most therapists have had to rely on less expensive and more accessible methods of measuring vestibular-ocular interaction. The most widely used clinical test is the Southern California Post-Rotary Nystagmus Test (SCPNT) developed by Ayres.[15] This test consists of rotating a child on a small turntable, stopping the turntable, and measuring the duration of the resulting nystagmus with a stopwatch. The SCPNT and its use with children is reviewed extensively in the following article of this volume.

Studies with learning disabled children have demonstrated, using the SCPNT, a correlation between a depressed nystagmus duration and poor postural mechanisms (i.e., hypotonia, poor prone extension, poor equilibrium reactions).[16,17] Although such a correlation may be real, no causative relationship should be assumed. Different CNS structures mediate different functions in vestibular-ocular and postural domains, and, although when one system is depressed, the other may also be depressed, this is not necessarily the case. Molina-Negro and associates, for example, in a study of 22 individuals with vertigo or disequilibrium, demonstrated no correlation between these subjects' performance on ENG tests and whether they had hyperactive or hypoactive postural reflexes.[18]

Wall and Black stated that vestibulo-ocular and vestibulo-spinal tests each assess a separate sensorimotor reflex of the vestibular system.[19] Because evidence exists that vestibular lesions can be localized in a small area of the vestibular end organs, only one of the two vestibular reflexes may be affected, however, lesions in the vestibular nuclei may affect both reflexes. These authors suggested that the use of just one type of test (i.e., either vestibular-ocular or postural) is not effective for screening for vestibular dysfunction.

Therapists should be concerned about some clinicians' reliance on nystagmus as an over-all indicator of vestibular function. If therapists were to perform only a tendon tap (a postural reflex) on a patient, what would it tell us about muscle tone or voluntary motor control? Not much! If we only test nystagmus (a vestibular-ocular reflex and small component of vestibular system circuitry) what does it tell us about the vestibular system? Again, possibly not much!

Normative Data

Normal nystagmus values have been obtained for various age-groups of children. Eviatar and co-workers used a torsion swing (perrotatory nystagmus) and ICC to test vestibular responses of 121 newborn infants.[20] The majority of appropriate for gestational age (AGA) babies demonstrated a response within the first 20 to 30 days of life. Perrotatory (torsion swing) and ICC vestibular stimulation were also used to study the nystagmus responses of 276 normal children.[13] Tests were administered at 3 month intervals from birth until 12 months of age and at 6 month intervals from 12 to 24 months of age. Within this age span, premature and small for gestational age (SGA) infants (as compared to AGA and large for gestational age LGA infants) demonstrated lower frequency, amplitude, speed of the slow component, and longer latency nystagmus responses during the first six months of life. Normative data from 0 to 24 months of age were presented which the authors suggested could be used to differentiate normal from abnormal responses.

Ornitz and co-workers rotated 46 normal children ranging in age from 1 month to 11 years at 10 degrees/second^2 for 18 seconds, then at a constant velocity of 180 degrees/second for 200 seconds in darkness.[21] ENG recordings of nystagmus were made and the data indicated a tendency for nystagmus parameters to decrease with increasing age. In addition, the ratio of slow component velocity of the secondary to primary nystagmus was greater in early infancy than at older ages.

Using an air caloric test, Andrieu-Guitrancourt and colleagues tested 140 normal children from 2 to 10 years of age.[22] The 4 and 5 year old children had increased nystagmus frequency as compared to those who were 2 and 3 years old, and the 8 to 10 year old children had increased nystagmus frequency as compared to those who were 6 and 7 years old. With increasing age, frequency of nystagmus beats increased, but maximum eye speed in the slow phase decreased.

In Tibbling's study of perrotatory nystagmus during constant velocity rotation in 84 normal children from newborn to 15 years of age, she found that the speed of the slow component, speed of the fast component, and amplitude decreased with increasing age.[10]

Several researchers have published normative nystagmus data for children of various ages using the SCPNT and these studies have been reviewed elsewhere.[23] In test-retest situations, the SCPNT has been demonstrated to be reliable for normal children.[15,24] In one study, reliability measures with learning-disabled children were lower than those established for normal children.[25] The validity of using the SCPNT with special populations is now beginning to be studied. Potter and Silverman demonstrated that a large percentage of children with sensorineural hearing loss (without handicapping conditions) have hypoactive vestibular responses.[26] Although many of the deaf children had poor static balance skills, balance was not significantly related to vestibular function as measured by the SCPNT.

POSTURAL TESTS

Neurophysiological Rationale

Several descending vestibular tracts are involved in postural control. Of the two direct descending routes from the vestibular nuclei, the medial vestibulospinal tract (MVST) is a smaller pathway which travels down the ventral white columns and ends in the cervical and upper thoracic segments of the spinal cord. The MVST is assumed to play a role in "adjustment of tone in neck muscles and regulation of head position".[27(p82)] In addition, the MVST may assist in coordinating head and eye movements and upper extremity balance reactions. The lateral vestibulospinal tract (LVST) is a larger ipsilateral tract which synapses at all levels of the spinal cord and is generally excitatory to extensor motorneurons and inhibitory to flexor motorneurons. The facilitory relationship between the LVST and extensor motorneurons is logical if the role of extensor muscles in maintaining anti-gravity postures is considered. Some reticulospinal fibers, however, are part of indirect pathways from the vestibular nuclei via the reticular system to the spinal cord and are excitatory to flexor and inhibitory to extensor motorneurons. The vestibular system is, therefore, able to act reciprocally on both flexors and extensors.

Vestibular input has been shown to elicit a response in both alpha and gamma motorneurons in human subjects. Some research indicates that the gamma motorneurons have a lower threshold for natural labyrinthine stimulation.[28] Generally, when vestibular stimulation occurs, preparation for execution of movement occurs and one component of this preparation may be a non-specific general enhancement of muscle tone.

Aiello and co-workers used the H-reflex to study the influence of different body tilts on the excitability of soleus alpha motorneurons in adults.[29] Ten normal subjects demonstrated a significant increase in amplitude of the H-reflex as the body was tilted from a horizontal to a vertical position and a decrease in amplitude of the H-reflex when returned to the horizontal position. No significant changes in H-reflex amplitude were noted in the one labyrinthine-defective individual who participated in the study. Visual and somatosensory inputs were removed or minimized, with the exception of somatosensory influences arising from weight distribution when subjects were moved on the platform. The results suggested that the vestibular system influences anti-gravity muscles during static tilts in an attempt to counteract gravity.

Vestibular input does not contribute isolated or sufficient information to control human posture. In particular, somatosensory, visual, and auditory stimuli interact with vestibular input to form integrated sensory signals. The vestibular nuclei also have complex interactions with other central nervous system structures. For example, one intimate interaction is with the cerebellum. Phylogenetically, the cerebellum evolved out of a primitive vestibular system and a close functional relationship remains between these two areas of the brain.[30] Ito has described a number of feedback loops between the vestibular nuclei and the cerebellum which are essential for both postural and ocular functions.[31] For example, head movement leads to compensatory eye movement (the VOR), however, receptors in the labyrinth cannot detect visual stimuli to determine if the eye movements were appropriate. Visual input to the flocculus travels to the vestibular nuclei and is used as an error signal to modulate vestibular-ocular reflexes. Similarly, when extremity righting reactions are needed to offset a loss of balance, receptors in the inner ear cannot monitor limb movements. Ascending somatosensory input from the posterior columns via the spinocerebellar tracts to the anterior lobe of the cerebellum and eventually to the vestibular nuclei provide the feedback necessary to determine if the postural response was appropriate.

Ascending pathways from all four vestibular nuclei are relayed to the cerebral cortex.[32] Although specific pathways have not been identified, the ventral posterolateral nucleus of the thalamus is thought to be one major relay center and additional long ascending pathways to the cortex via the cerebellum and reticular formation have been proposed. The critical point is that information in ascending vestibular pathways does not consist of isolated signals from the peripheral vestibular organ, but is already a complex signal receiving multiple sensory inputs regarding motion and posture.[33] In particular, somatosensory and vestibular information are processed in an integrated fashion.

The bilateral representation of somatosensory and vestibular information exists all the way to the cerebral cortex where the primary association areas for vestibular input are not solely for vestibular signals, but also for somatosensory input.[34,35] This duality of information is unique in the cortex where other sensory inputs have single primary association areas.

Methodological Considerations

The contrast in the level of description of vestibular postural reflexes as compared to vestibular-ocular tests is marked. The relative lack of progress in devising vestibular postural assessments may be "due to the fact that in normal, real-life situations, vestibular effects are subsumed into complex postural responses which reflect also sensory information of other modalities (visual, somatic, and proprioceptive), all of which are likely to strongly interact with each other".[36(p413)] Uemura and associates provide an excellent review of vestibular postural tests which are currently used in medical diagnostic procedures.[37] Physicians who administer these tests are usually interested in detecting labyrinthine disorders, such as Meniere's disease, labyrinthitis, vestibular neuronitis, and acoustic neuroma. Therapists, however, are often administering postural tests to study more subtle and complex central nervous system disturbances. For this reason, although some of the same tests are administered, therapists also assess postural functions not usually included by otolaryngologists in typical test administration.

Two classic vestibular postural tests include Fukada's stepping and writing tests, which are based on the premise that a vestibular deficit will be revealed by relative loss of postural tone or the inability to produce normal muscle tension on the ipsilateral side of the body as compared to the contralateral side.[38,39] In the stepping test, the subject is asked to close his eyes and raise his hands above his head, then to mark time (i.e., 50 steps) in the center of the circle. Departures from the center of the circle or circular deviations are calculated. If, for example, a lesion exists in the inner ear or vestibular nuclei on the right side extensor muscles on the right side of the body will have less activity and relatively greater extension will be produced on the left side. This "stronger" left side will cause the subject to deviate toward the right.

In one study of 40 normal adults, using a modified stepping test, the mean rotation of 23 of the 40 subjects was between 30 and 60 degrees and forward movement in 22 subjects was between 50 and 100 cm.[40] The authors concluded that the great variability between subjects and within individuals from one test to another made the stepping test of little diagnostic importance. According to Uemura and associates, however, "body rotation of more than 30 degrees, backward displacement of the final position or forward displacement of more than 1 meter are regarded as abnormal".[37(p32)] In the writing test, the subject sits in a chair in front of a desk with a pencil in the dominant hand (other hand on knee). The subject writes 4 or 5 large capital alphabetical letters vertically on graph paper with the arm fully extended and with neither the arm nor body touching the desk. This procedure is carried out with the eyes open and the eyes closed. "If a deviation of more than 10 degrees is found solely in the letters written during the blindfold test, unilateral labyrinthine lesion may be indicated".[37(p34)]

Pavlov and Irintchev compared performance on Fukada's tests to complete otoneurological examinations, including ENG testing, in 115 subjects with varying vestibular related diagnoses and 35 normal control subjects.[41] The results indicated that Fukada's tests were of diagnostic importance, especially in the acute stages of labyrinthine disorders. However, because one-third of the control group demonstrated deviations with both tests, it was concluded that these tests must be combined with additional diagnostic methods.

Another routine clinical postural test which has been used is the Romberg—or standing with eyes closed. Black and Wall demonstrated that this test is of questionable clinical value for detecting vestibular disorders, as patients with intact proprioceptive systems can compensate well enough to perform this postural task in spite of vestibular deficits.[42] Baloh and Honrubia agreed that the Romberg is not a sensitive test, but stated that the "sharpened Romberg" (patient is in a heel-to-toe position with eyes closed, arms folded across chest) is a more demanding measure of balance . . . "normal subjects can stand in this position for 30 seconds, while patients with unilateral or bilateral vestibular impairment rarely can sustain the position".[43(p107)]

Dynamic postural tests such as tandem walking with eyes open and eyes closed put a greater demand on the vestibular system than do static tests. Normative data for tandem walking or "Walk on Floor Eyes Closed" (WOFEC) were obtained for male and female children at 8, 10, 12, 14, 16, and 18 years by Cunningham and Goetzinger.[44] Clyse and Short demonstrated significant relationships between WOFEC, nystagmus duration, Walk on Floor Eyes Open, age, muscle tone, and standing balance with the eyes open in a group of learning disabled children and suggested that dynamic balance should be included with other clinical variables in the evaluation of vestibular function.[17]

deQuiros and Schrager described use of a changing-consistency board to examine vestibular-proprioceptive functions in children.[45] A changing-consistency board looks like a solid wooden board, but at one point its consistency is abruptly changed from a hard to a soft surface. The subject's vision cannot provide him with information regarding the change of consistency because the surface of the board looks consistent. deQuiros and Schrager stated that when the subject suddenly steps on the soft part of the board, vestibular and other postural systems (i.e., proprioceptive, tactile and visual) must be employed to maintain balance.

Uemura and associates discussed the ramifications of imbalance between labyrinths on equilibrium functions.[37] If an individual with left labyrinthine damage is asked to stand with the eyes closed and the arms extended forward, a characteristic posture called the "discus-thrower" position may be observed. In this condition the eyes deviate (slow phase) to the left with spontaneous nystagmus (quick phase) to the right. Head turning and trunk twisting to the left may occur with deviation of both arms to the left accompanied by raising of the right arm and lowering of the left arm. The patient may also demonstrate a tendency to fall and a deviation of gait to the left. Following labyrinthectomy, non-human mammals consistently develop marked ipsilateral hypotonia in extensor muscles. Baloh and Honrubia stated that although a similar degree of hypotonia is not usually observed in human subjects, a slight asymmetry in posture with the ipsilateral arm slightly flexed and abducted compared to the contralateral arm may be noted.[42] Deep tendon reflexes, those which are usually elicited clinically, are also unaffected by vestibular lesions. Apparently other supraspinal influences compensate for the loss of vestibular signals. According to Uemura and associates, bilateral labyrinthine damage, which is fairly equal in extent, "may appear as a disturbance of the righting reflex, i.e., an unsteadiness of the body in all directions".[37(p32)]

Past-pointing is another postural test often used to assess imbalance of the vestibular system. The subject extends the upper extremity with his index finger on the index finger of the examiner. With eyes closed, the subject raises his arm to a vertical position and then returns it to the examiner's finger. Constant deviation to one side (usually toward the side of the vestibular deficit) may indicate a vestibular related impairment.

More sophisticated postural analyses have been developed by researchers (unfortunately, not yet applicable to clinical settings) in recent years. One technique involves force platforms with strain gauges "whose signals are combined by computer and displayed as a moving vector indicating the point of application, magnitude and direction of the resultant contact force between the feet and the ground".[46(p397)] Analyses of resulting data can provide information on standing balance in normal subjects and patterns of abnormality in different disorders.

What postural tests do physical and occupational therapists currently use to assess vestibular function in the pediatric client? In many clinical settings the therapist uses a battery of postural tasks, including the ability of the child to assume and maintain a prone extension pattern against gravity, to produce appropriate righting and equilibrium responses, and to inhibit the use of the tonic neck reflexes.

The ability to assume and maintain a totally extended posture against gravity (Figure 1) is hypothesized to require adequate processing of gravity information via the vestibular nuclei (particularly Deiters' nucleus), down the LVST to extensor motorneurons. Ayres discussed the prone extension posture in relation to the role of the gravity receptors and neck proprioceptors. She stated that motion when the child is resting on the abdomen is an effective stimulus for eliciting trunk extension.[47] Harris demonstrated, in a normative study, that the performance of 4 year old children varied considerably on this task, but that by six years of age, children should be able not only to assume the prone extension posture, but to maintain it for 30 seconds.[48]

Righting reactions and equilibrium responses can be tested by lifting the child in space or changing the child's position while on a variety of moveable surfaces. Lateral tilt, for example, activates utricular receptors which in turn excite vestibulospinal neurons and influence the activity of limb muscles.[49] In theory, use of a blindfold in testing can eliminate visual influences, however, many normal children do not tolerate being blindfolded and then placed in situations where their balance is challenged. Children with balance deficits are even less tolerant of being blindfolded. Age guidelines for head righting, equilibrium responses and other postural reactions which are dependent, at least in part, on vestibular processing have been documented by many developmental researchers,[4,50,51] and are well-known to therapists who work in pediatrics.

Another clinical observation relates to the presence of tonic neck postures. Problems in integration of tonic neck reflexes may implicate related vestibular dysfunction because labyrinthine receptors indicate body position only in conjunction with neck receptors. A close examination of the effects on the extremities of the tonic neck reflexes and the labyrinthine righting reflexes demonstrates that these two postural mech-

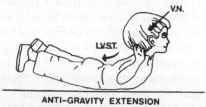

ANTI-GRAVITY EXTENSION

FIGURE 1. The vestibular nuclei (VN) contribute to anti-gravity extension by activation of extensor muscles of the trunk and proximal joints via the lateral vestibulospinal tract (LVST).

anisms elicit exactly opposite changes in postural tone[52] (Figure 2). The common description of the ATNR as producing increased extensor tone on the face side and increased flexor tone on the skull side is not technically correct. A more precise definition would be that increased extensor tone is produced on the face side, and less extensor tone is elicited on the skull side with resulting flexion.

In phylogenetically early animals who did not have a neck (i.e., fish) the vestibular apparatus was sufficient for determining body position. In animals who developed the ability to move the head on the body, vestibular input was no longer sufficient to monitor body position. For example, in Figure 3, if the CNS has only information from the labyrinthine receptors, it cannot tell whether the head has moved on the body or the body has moved in space, as the vestibular input is the same. In Condition A, neck receptors inform the CNS that the head has moved on the body (not the body through space); in Condition B, the neck receptors inform the CNS that the head has not moved on the body (therefore, the body must have moved through space). These two sets of postural responses work together as a functional unit and abnormal reliance or posturing related to one component may affect the efficiency of processing by the other component. The dual representation of somatosensory and vestibular information throughout the central nervous system should now be more logical as the CNS needs both elements of information for postural, ocular and spatial orientation functions. It also explains Fukada's rationale for varying the administration of his writing and stepping tests to blindfolded subjects by turning the head to one side in order to determine the "expression of the tonic neck reflexes".[39(p17)]

A clinical evaluation of vestibular function would not be complete without a judgment of muscle tone. Although disagreement exists as to whether muscle tone is a critical issue in developmental assessment,[53] muscle tone is closely associated with the integrity of the vestibular system.[54] Vestibular end organs contain a high proportion of units from which impulse activity can be recorded even in the absence of stimulation. This "resting discharge" plays an integral part in vestibular function and the labyrinth must be considered one of the most important sources of general muscle tonus. "The resting discharge furnishes a continuous influx of 'excitation' via the vestibular nuclei into the motor centers associated with postural and locomotory muscle systems".[54(p101)] Loss of vestibular input may result in prolonged muscular debility that may even extend to visceral muscles.

The unclear delineation between muscle tension at rest (due to neural control, viscoelasticity inherent in the muscle, its tendon, surrounding connective tissues, and the fibrous tissues around the joint)[55] and the ability to generate muscle tension in appropriate movement patterns is probably a contributing factor to the ambiguous concept of muscle "tone".

Muscle tone is often analyzed through palpation of muscle bulk and visual observation of resting posture in a variety of positions relative to gravity (i.e., supine, prone, standing). Fukada's tests, the Romberg, tandem walking, past-pointing, prone extension, and righting and equilibrium reactions reflect the ability to generate appropriate muscle tension in correct temporal patterns. Both elements (resting tension and generation of movement) may be related to vestibular dysfunction but, in my clinical experience, are not necessarily predictive of each other.

Implications for the Clinician

The unfortunate reality of the study of the vestibular system is that it is too simplistic to study sensory systems or motor responses in isolation.

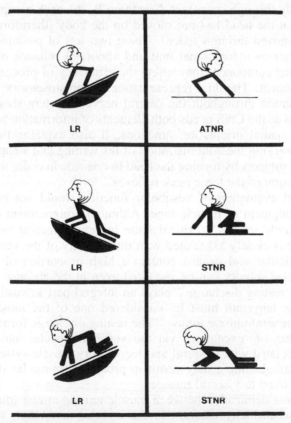

FIGURE 2. Labyrinthine righting (LR) and tonic neck (ATNR & STNR) responses produce opposite effects on the extremities. For example, in quadruped when the body (and head) is tilted down, the arms extend and the hips flex. When the head flexes on the trunk, the arms flex and the hips extend (bottom figures).

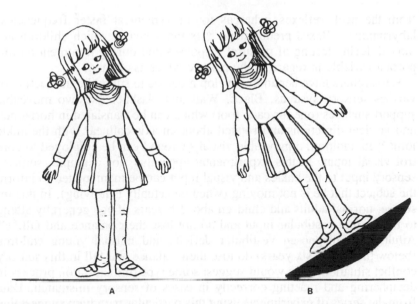

A   B

FIGURE 3. If the body is tilted (B) or the head moved on the trunk (A) in the same plane of motion
with identical excursion and rate of movement, the labyrinths receive the same stimulus. Information
from neck receptors provide the CNS with information to determine whether the body has moved in
space or the head has moved on the body. Body proprioception, signalling the presence or absence of
weight-shift, and visual input also contribute to the orientation process.

We must begin to consider and to study the complex interactions that
typify human sensory processing and movement. For example, various
authors suggested that the "parachute reaction" (forward protective extension) was either a visual or a vestibular mediated response. Wenzel
demonstrated that to obtain the optimal response, *both* visual and vestibular information were necessary.[56] We need to change our perception of
"vestibular" assessment to encompass the dynamic flexibility of inter-
sensory integration which may vary depending upon the environmental
context of the task.

Although the role of the ATNR in eye-hand coordination has face validity, this relationship may have been imposed on what is, in reality, part
of the postural response system. Consider how long the infant and young
child must rely on and integrate information from the labyrinths and neck
receptors as postural control is developed in prone, on hands and knees,
and in standing. Not a single developmental study has addressed the interaction of vestibular and proprioceptive systems in postural control. The
relationship between these two sets of postural responses may also be
critical in terms of clinical test procedures and treatment. Anderson and
co-workers stated that movement at low frequencies, as a static position is
approached, results in a predominance of motor output to limb extensors

from the neck reflexes, whereas for movement at faster frequencies, labyrinthine reflexes predominate.[36] Is the speed at which children are moved during testing of postural responses and during treatment an important variable in regard to the posture which is elicited?

Researchers have begun to develop methods to study the interaction of various sensory systems. Black, Wall and Nashner use two moveable support surfaces (one for each foot) which can be translated in horizontal and vertical directions and rotated about an axis colinear with the ankle joint.[57] In addition, a moveable visual surround can be employed to control visual input. In this experimental apparatus, for example, somatosensory input to the ankles and visual input can be manipulated to inform the subject that he is not moving (when he actually is moving). In this instance, normal adults and children above 6 years of age generally attend to the correct vestibular input and do not lose their balance and fall.[58,59] Adults with diagnosed vestibular deficits and normal young children (below the age of six years) do lose their balance and fall in this sensory conflict situation. This would suggest some type of maturation process in deciphering and reacting correctly in cases of sensory mismatch. Data from the series of experiments using this particular paradigm suggest that one major function of the vestibular system may be to resolve sensory conflicts, especially as the process of inter-sensory integration may relate to motor control.

The complex interaction of sensory integration and motor control has also been studied in children with diagnosed brain dysfunction.[60] Children with varying diagnoses of cerebral palsy (ataxia, athetosis, spastic diplegia, spastic hemiplegia) performed differently when their posture was destabilized by sensory conflicts compared to their ability to produce normal muscle coordination.

Another approach has been to study the process of compensation for vestibular deficiencies. Bles and co-workers used a tilting room and reported the postural and perceptual responses of normal, uni- and bilaterally labyrinthless subjects to sinusoidal lateral tilting of the visual surround.[61] The subjects stood on a stabilometer which measured body sway. As in Nashner and Black's research, normal subjects used correct somatosensory and vestibular input rather than misleading visual stimuli. Labyrinthless patients initially relied on vision alone and did not report room movement, but perceived, incorrectly, platform movement and, therefore, exhibited marked postural swaying. After a period of time, labyrinthless subjects regained postural stability and correctly perceived the room as moving. The authors suggested that this compensation reflected an increase in the relative weight imparted to the somatic afferent system in this task. This apparent dynamic flexibility of sensory integration is encouraging in terms of the possible efficacy of intervention techniques.

Normative Data

In regard to postural tests, some data relevant to testing children have been accumulated. Various tests of standing balance with eyes open and eyes closed and of tandem walking are part of larger test batteries.[62,63]

Selected items on some standardized tests, such as the Miller Assessment of Preschoolers and the Southern California Sensory Integration Tests can be considered to tap vestibular functions.[62,64] DeGangi and co-workers developed a battery of vestibular-based tests for pre-school children (3-5 years) and Dunn published normative data on vestibular-related postural responses in kindergarten children.[65,66] As clinicians, however, we do not have normative data on a vestibular postural test battery, validated on vestibular-defective children, to use for patient comparison, such as Fregley's Ataxia Test Battery for adults.[67] In addition, further research and adaptation of current methods of studying intersensory processes are necessary for clinical assessment of vestibular postural functions in children to become not only feasible, but also relevant to intervention programs.

DEVELOPMENTAL CONSIDERATIONS

Several studies of infant nystagmus using caloric stimulation, torsion swings, and rotatory stimulation, have demonstrated that the presence of a nystagmus response along with birthweight are important indices to CNS maturation.[20,68] Tonic eye deviations (the slow or vestibular component) can be elicited immediately following birth, and nystagmus (both slow and fast components) usually appears within the first month for AGA infants and within 3 to 4 months for SGA infants. A delayed nystagmus response is usually seen in the premature infant.

We have little information about the possible ramifications of vestibular deficits on the development and use of the VOR in children. Only recently have researchers demonstrated that adults in acute stages of labyrinthine disorders have impaired ability to fixate visually on a stationary target with natural head movements.[69]

The effect of arousal on the nystagmus response has been studied extensively in adults and has also been documented in newborn infants and children.[70,71] In fact, the failure or ability to elicit caloric nystagmus is such a valid indicator of brain stem function, that this test has been used to corroborate diagnoses of brain death.[72]

Fish and Dixon, in a longitudinal study of ten infants born to schizophrenic mothers, suggested that the transitory nature of depressed nystagmus responses ruled out the possibility of an organic lesion in the vestibular system, per se, but was probably the result of transitory decreases in the arousal system.[73] Perhaps therapists should turn their research efforts and clinical attention to determining if nystagmus could be used clinically as a measure of arousal rather than as a measure of vestibular function.

An important consideration for therapists when analyzing reactions to stimuli or behavioral responses in assessment and treatment is the "state" of the individual. Brazelton observed that reactions to stimuli may vary markedly as the infant passes from one behavioral state to another.[74] Disorders of arousal and attention are also well documented in children with brain dysfunction.[75] Measures of bodily changes[76] could be compared to nystagmus responses under similar conditions of arousal and attention to determine if nystagmus could be used as a clinical measure of arousal.

Few studies have been made of the early functioning of the vestibulospinal system. In one study of the newborn postural system what appeared to be constant vestibulospinal control at a few hours following birth was demonstrated.[77] In that study EMG records of stretch reflexes were used which were affected by movement of the infant while lying on a platform (linear and vertical accelerations and decelerations). Both inhibitory and excitatory influences on the motorneuron pool were noted.

Some developmental implications may be related to the close functional relationship between the vestibular nuclei and the cerebellum. Erway stated that "the vestibular system, especially the otoliths, may be uniquely important among all of the sensory organs in the development of normal integrative functions of the brain, especially the cerebellum" . . . and on this basis—can argue "that any genetic or environmental factors which alter the normal development or maintenance of this elaborate inertial-guidance system may affect the development of early locomotor functions."[78(p24)]

Connolly and Michael suggested a relationship between the side of elicited ATNR and convexity of the scoliotic curve in children.[79] When the ATNR was elicited with the face to the left, the convexity of the curve was also on the left. This result would fit with a hypothesis suggested by Nachemson and Sahlstrand, that a unilateral vestibular deficit would result in an asymmetry in postural tone where the individual would lean and rotate toward the side of least tonicity and the spine would, therefore, demonstrate a lateral deviation and rotation—or scoliosis.[80] The results of Connolly and Michael's study are logical when, again, one considers the relationship between the tonic neck reflexes and the labyrinthine reflexes acting on the extremities and trunk.

The developmental implications of vestibular deficits are unclear because we are unable to identify vestibular dysfunction in a precise manner, particularly in the infant and young child. The human vestibular apparatus, however, is known to be susceptible to traumatic injuries and to genetic defects. Wright with colleagues, in two post-mortem studies, examined the inner ears of 31 fetuses from 14 to 36 weeks gestation and of

30 infants from birth to two years of age.[81,82] Maturation of labyrinthine structures continued after birth and because some detached membranes were noted, they suggested that the inner ear is susceptible to pathology and trauma in infancy. Wright and colleagues, in a case study of a 6 week old infant with several congenital abnormalities, demonstrated on autopsy that the infant had no otoconia bilaterally.[83] Steel and Bock defined a classification scheme for inner-ear abnormalities in animals with hereditary inner-ear defects and discussed the relevance of this classification scheme to conditions in humans.[84]

When researchers are able to diagnose vestibular deficits in a much more precise manner in infancy, longitudinal studies of the development of these children can be undertaken. One is tempted to hypothesize that infants born with severe genetic abnormalities or who are subjected to severe trauma of the vestibular receptors will have major developmental problems. One might assume with equal logic, however, that because the vestibular system interacts with so many other sensory systems, the probability of compensation and resulting normal function is high. Other components of the vestibular system may compensate for absence or non-functioning of the inner ear vestibular end organs.

Sensory integrative deficits of the CNS will be even more difficult to diagnose and study longitudinally in children. Vestibular compensation has been studied in adults with varying diagnoses.[85] Pfaltz stated that vestibular compensation is accomplished through a multisensory substitution process in an actively behaving individual. He also suggested the possibility of "an early critical period during which adaptive changes are induced by multisensory inputs."[85(p405)] What implications the process of compensation in adults has for the treatment of children with vestibular dysfunction or anomalies is unknown but is certainly an area of importance for the clinician.

In summary, the assessment of vestibular function is complex and may best be accomplished within a framework involving multiple sensory and motor systems and specific environmental or behavioral tasks. The challenge for occupational and physical therapists is to continually incorporate changing theoretical constructs and models of vestibular assessment and function into clinical practice while the neurosciences provide us with data and, hopefully, guidelines for the study of our clinically-related questions.

REFERENCES

1. Highstein SM, Reisine H: Synaptic and functional organization of vestibulo-ocular reflex pathways, in Granit R, Pompeiano O (eds): *Reflex Control of Posture and Movement. Progress in Brain Research*, New York, Elsevier/North-Holland Biomedical Press, 1979, vol 50, pp 431-442.

2. Barber HO, Stockwell CW: *Manual of Electronystagmography*. St Louis, CV Mosby Company, 1976.

3. Yee RD, Baloh RW, Honrubia V, Kim YS: A study of congenital nystagmus: Vestibular nystagmus. *J Otolaryngol* 10:89-98, 1981.

4. Eviatar L, Eviatar A: Neurovestibular examination of infants and children. *Adv Otorhinolaryngol* 23:169-191, 1978.

5. Holsopple JQ: Factors affecting the duration of post-rotation nystagmus. *J Comp Physiol Psychol* 3:283-304, 1923.

6. Pfaltz CR: Quantitative parameters in nystagmography. *J Oto-Rhino-Laryngol* 36:46-52, 1974.

7. Johnson DD, Torok N: Habituation of nystagmus and sensation of motion after rotation. *Acta Otolaryngol (Stockh)* 69:206-215, 1970.

8. Henriksson NG: The correlation between the speed of the eye in the slow phase of nystagmus and vestibular stimulus. *Acta Otolaryngol (Stockh)* 42:120-136, 1955.

9. Torok N: Nystagmus frequency versus slow phase velocity in rotatory and caloric nystagmus. *Ann Otol Rhinol Laryngol* 78:625-640, 1969.

10. Tibbling L: The rotatory nystagmus response in children. *Acta Otolaryngol (Stockh)* 68:459-467, 1969.

11. Henriksson NG: Speed of slow component and duration in caloric nystagmus. *Acta Otolaryngol (Suppl)* 125:1-29, 1956.

12. Hyden D, Larsby BK, Schwarz DWF, Odkvist LM: Quantification of slow compensatory eye movements in patients with bilateral vestibular loss. *Acta Otolaryngol* 96:199-206, 1983.

13. Eviatar L, Eviatar A: The normal nystagmic response of infants to caloric and perrotatory stimulation. *Laryngoscope* 89:1036-1045, 1979.

14. McCabe BF: Part V. Experimental methods in vestibular research, in Smith CA, Vernon JA (eds): *Handbook of Auditory and Vestibular Research Methods*. Springfield, IL, Charles C Thomas, 1976.

15. Ayres AJ: *Southern California Post-rotary Nystagmus Test*. Los Angeles, Western Psychological Services, 1975.

16. Ottenbacher K: Identifying vestibular processing dysfunction in learning disabled children. *Am J Occup Ther* 32:217-221, 1978.

17. Clyse SJ, Short MA: The relationship between dynamic balance and postrotary nystagmus in learning disabled children. *Phys Occup Ther Pediatr* 3:25-32, 1983.

18. Molina-Negro P, Bertrand RA, Matine E, Gioani Y: The role of the vestibular system in relation to muscle tone and postural reflexes in man. *Acta Otolaryngol (Stockh)* 89:524-533, 1980.

19. Wall C, Black FO: Postural stability and rotational tests: Their effectiveness for screening dizzy patients. *Acta Otolaryngol (Stockh)* 95:235-246, 1983.

20. Eviatar L, Eviatar A, Naray I: Maturation of neurovestibular responses in infants. *Dev Med Child Neurol* 16:435-446, 1974.

21. Ornitz EM, Atwell CW, Walter DO, et al.: The maturation of vestibular nystagmus in infancy and childhood. *Acta Otolaryngol* 88:244-256, 1979.

22. Andrieu-Guitrancourt J, Peron JM, Dehesdin D, et al.: Normal vestibular responses to air caloric tests in children. *Int J Pediatr Oto-rhinolaryngol* 3:245-250, 1981.

23. Crowe TK, Deitz JC, Siegner CB: Postrotatory nystagmus response of normal four-year-old children. *Phys Occup Ther Pediatr* 4:19-28, 1984.

24. Kimball J: Normative comparison of the Southern California Postrotary Nystagmus Test: Los Angeles vs. Syracuse data. *Am J Occup Ther* 35:21-25, 1981.

25. Morrison D, Sublett J: Reliability of the Southern California Postrotary Nystagmus Test with learning disabled children. *Am J Occup Ther* 37:694-698, 1983.

26. Potter CN, Silverman LN: Characteristics of vestibular function and static balance skills in deaf children. *Phys Ther* 64:1071-1075, 1984.

27. Nyberg-Hansen R: Anatomical aspects of the functional organization of the vestibulospinal pathways, in Naunton RF (ed): *The Vestibular System*, New York, Academic Press, 1975, pp 71-96.

28. Gantchev GN, Draganova N: Vestibular influences upon spinal (H and T) reflexes in man. *Agressologie* 19:39-40, 1978.

29. Aiello I, Rosati G, Serra G, et al.: Static vestibulospinal influences in relation to different body tilts in man. *Exp Neurol* 79:18-26, 1983.

30. Sarnat HB, Netsky MG: Vestibular and acoustic system, in *Evolution of the Nervous System*. New York, Oxford Press, 1974, chapter 5.

31. Ito M: The vestibulo-cerebellar relationships: Vestibulo-ocular reflex arc and flocculus, in Naunton RF (ed): *The Vestibular System*, New York, Academic Press, 1975, pp 129-146.

32. Blum PS, Abraham LD, Gilman S: Vestibular, auditory and somatic input to the posterior thalamus of the cat. *Exp Brain Res* 34:1-9, 1979.

33. Buttner U, Lang W: The vestibulocortical pathway: neurophysiological and anatomical studies in the monkey, in Granit R, Pompeiano O (eds): *Reflex Control of Posture and Movement. Progress in Brain Research*, New York, Elsevier/North-Holland Biomedical Press, 1979, vol 50, pp 581-588.

34. Odkvist LM, Liedgran SRC, Larsby B, Jerlvall L: Vestibular and somatosensory inflow to the vestibular projection area in the posterior cruciate dimple region of the cat cerebral cortex. *Exp Brain Res* 22:185-196, 1975.

35. Schwarz DWF, Fredrickson JM: Rhesus monkey vestibular cortex: A bimodal primary projection field. *Science* 172:280-281, 1971.

36. Anderson JH, Soechting JF, Terzuolo CA: Role of vestibular inputs in the organization of motor output to forelimb extensors, in Granit R, Pompeiano O (eds): *Reflex Control of Posture and Movement, Progress in Brain Research*, New York, Elsevier/North-Holland Biomedical Press, 1979, vol 50, pp 413-421.

37. Uemura T, Suzuki J, Hozawa J, Highstein S: *Neuro-otological Examination with Special Reference to Equilibrium Function Tests*. Baltimore, University Park Press, 1977.

38. Fukada T: Vertical writing with eyes covered: A new test of vestibulospinal reaction. *Acta Otolaryngol (Stockh)* 50:26-36, 1959.

39. Fukada T: Studies on human dynamic postures from the viewpoint of postural reflexes. *Acta Otolaryngol (Suppl)* 161:1-52, 1961.

40. Zilstorff-Pedersen K, Peitersen E: Vestibulospinal reflexes. I. Spontaneous alterations in the position of normal persons doing the stepping test. *Arch Otolaryngol* 77:237-242, 1963.

41. Pavlov DD, Irintchev E: Fukada writing and stepping tests in the evaluation of vestibular disturbances in labyrinth diseases. *Agressologie* 19(B):71-72, 1978.

42. Black FO, Wall C III: Comparison of vestibulo-ocular and vestibulo-spinal screening tests. *Otolaryngol Head Neck Surg* 89:811-817, 1981.

43. Baloh RW, Honrubia V: *Clinical Neurophysiology of the Vestibular System*. Philadelphia, Davis Company, 1979.

44. Cunningham DR, Goetzinger CP. Floor ataxia test battery. *Arch Otolaryngol* 96:559-564, 1972.

45. deQuiros JB, Schrager OL: *Neuropsychological Fundamentals in Learning Disabilities*. San Rafael, CA, Academic Therapy, 1978.

46. Roberts TDM, Stenhouse G: Reactions to overbalancing, in Granit R, Pompeiano O (eds): *Reflex Control of Posture and Movement, Progress in Brain Research*, New York, Elsevier/North-Holland Biomedical Press, 1979, vol 50, pp 397-404.

47. Ayres AJ: *Sensory Integration and Learning Disorders*. Los Angeles, Western Psychological Services, 1973.

48. Harris NP: Duration and quality of the prone extension position in four, six and eight year old normal children. *Am J Occup Ther* 35:26-30, 1981.

49. Maeda M: Semicircular canal and macular influences on neck motorneurons, in Granit R, Pompeiano O (eds): *Reflex Control of Posture and Movement, Progress in Brain Research*, New York, Elsevier/North-Holland Biomedical Press, 1979, vol 50, pp 405-412.

50. Paine RS, Brazelton B, Donovan DE, et al.: Evolution of postural reflexes in normal infants and in the presence of chronic brain syndrome. *Neurology* 14:1036-1048, 1964.

51. Peiper A: Reflexes of position and movement, in *Cerebral Function in Infancy and Childhood*. New York, Consultants Bureau, 1963, pp 147-210.

52. Rosenberg JR, Lindsay KW: Asymmetric tonic labyrinthine reflexes. *Brain Res* 63: 347-350, 1973.

53. Milani-Comparetti A: Pattern analysis of normal and abnormal development: The fetus, the newborn, the child, in Slaton DS (ed): *Development of Movement in Infancy*. Chapel Hill, NC, University of North Carolina at Chapel Hill, 1981, pp 1-33.

54. Lowenstein O: The peripheral neuron, in Naunton RF (ed): *The Vestibular System*, New York, Academic Press, 1975, pp 99-107.

55. Myers GJ: Understanding the floppy baby, in Griggs RC, Moxley RT (eds): *Advances in Neurology*. New York, Raven Press, 1977, vol 17, pp 295-315.

56. Wenzel D: The development of the parachute reaction: A visuo-vestibular response. *Neuropadiatrie* 19:351-359, 1978.

57. Black FO, Wall C III, Nashner LM: Effects of visual and support surface orientation references upon postural control in vestibular deficient subjects. *Acta Otolaryngol (Stockh)* 95:199-210, 1983.

58. Forssberg H, Nashner LM: Ontogenetic development of postural control in man: Adaptation to altered support and visual conditions during stance. *J Neurosc* 2:545-552, 1982.

59. Nashner LM, Black FO, Wall C: Adaptation to altered support and visual conditions during stance: Patients with vestibular deficits. *J Neurosci* 2:536-544, 1982.

60. Nashner LM, Shumway-Cook A, Marin O. Stance posture control in select groups of children with cerebral palsy: Deficits in sensory organization and muscular coordination. *Exp Brain Res* 49:393-409, 1983.

61. Bles W, Vianney de Jong JMB, deWit G: Compensation for labyrinthine defects examined by use of a tilting room. *Acta Otolaryngol (Stockh)* 95:576-579, 1983.

62. Ayres AJ: *Southern California Sensory Integration Tests*, Los Angeles, Western Psychological Services, 1972.

63. Stott DH, Moyes FA, Henderson SE: *Test of Motor Impairment*, Guelph, Ontario, Brook Educational Publishing Ltd, 1984.

64. Miller L: *Miller Assessment for Preschoolers*. Littleton, CO. Foundation for Knowledge in Development, 1982.

65. DeGangi GA, Berk RA, Larsen LA: The measurement of vestibular-based functions in preschool children. *Am J Occup Ther* 34:452-459, 1980.

66. Dunn W: *A Guide to Testing Clinical Observations in Kindergartners*. Rockville, MD, American Occupational Therapy Association, 1981.

67. Fregley AR: Vestibular ataxia and its measurement in man, in Kornhuber HH (ed): *Handbook of Sensory Physiology, Vestibular System. Part 2: Psychophysics, Applied Aspects and General Interpretations*. New York, Springer-Verlag, 1974, pp 321-360.

68. Rossi LN, Pignataro O, Nino LM, et al.: Maturation of vestibular responses: Preliminary report. *Dev Med Child Neurol* 21:217-224, 1979.

69. Takahashi M, Uemura T, Fujishiro T: Compensatory eye movements and gaze fixation during active head rotation in patients with labyrinthine disorders. *Ann Otol Rhinol Laryngol* 90:241-245, 1981.

70. von Bernuth H, Prechtl HFR: Vestibulo-ocular response and its state dependency in newborn infants. *Neuropadiatrie* 1:11-24, 1969.

71. Montgomery PC, Capps MJ: Effect of arousal on the nystagmus response of normal children. *Phys Occup Ther Pediatr* 1:17-30, 1980.

72. Hicks RG, Torda TA: The vestibulo-ocular (caloric) reflex in the diagnosis of cerebral death. *Anaesthesia Int Care* 7:169-173, 1979.

73. Fish B, Dixon WJ: Vestibular hyporeactivity in infants at risk for schizophrenia. *Arch Gen Psychiatry* 35:963-971, 1978.

74. Brazelton TB: *Neonatal Behavioral Assessment Scale*. Clinics in Developmental Medicine, No 50. Philadelphia, JB Lippincott Co, 1973.

75. Rapin I: Disorders of attention and arousal, in *Children with Brain Dysfunction*. New York, Raven Press, 1982, pp 95-104.

76. Hugelin A: Bodily changes during arousal, attention and emotion, in Hockman CH (ed): *Limbic System Mechanisms and Autonomic Function*, Springfield, IL, Charles C Thomas, 1972, pp 202-219.

77. Antonova TG, Vakhrameeva IA: Vestibulospinal influences in early human postnatal development. *Neurosci Behav Physiol* 6:151-156, 1973.

78. Erway L: Otolith formation and trace elements: A theory of schizophrenic behavior. *J Orthomol Psychiatry* 4:16-26, 1975.

79. Connolly BH, Michael BT: Early detection of scoliosis: A neurological approach using the asymmetrical tonic neck reflex. *Phys Ther* 64:304-307, 1984.

80. Nachemson AL, Sahlstrand T: Etiologic factors in adolescent idiopathic scoliosis. *Spine* 2:176-183, 1977.

81. Wright CG, Hubbard DG, Clark G: Observations of human fetal otoconial membranes. *Ann Otol Rhinol Laryngol* 88:267-274, 1979.

82. Wright CG, Hubbard DG: Observations of otoconial membranes from human infants. *Acta Otolaryngol (Stockh)* 86:185-194, 1978.

83. Wright CG, Hubbard DG, Grahman JW: Absence of otoconia in a human infant. *Ann Otol Rhinol Laryngol* 88:779-783, 1979.

84. Steel KP, Bock GR: Hereditary inner-ear abnormalities in animals. *Arch Otolaryngol* 109: 22-29, 1983.

85. Pfaltz, CR: Vestibular compensation. *Acta Otolaryngol (Stockh)* 95:402-406, 1983.

Reliability and Clinical Significance of the Southern California Postrotary Nystagmus Test

Rebecca E. Dutton, MS, OTR

ABSTRACT. The purpose of this paper is to review the literature related to the reliability and clinical validity of the Southern California Postrotary Nystagmus Test. Extensive research has been done on both normal and abnormal school age children and on normal and high-risk infants. Precautions for administration and guidelines for interpretation of postrotary nystagmus test scores are discussed. Alternate methods of measuring nystagmus, such as caloric and per-rotary induced nystagmus, are compared to postrotary nystagmus.

INTRODUCTION

Ayres developed a standardized test called the *Southern California Postrotary Nystagmus Test* (SCPNT)[1] which was influential in introducing the evaluation of nystagmus to the field of occupational therapy. This test measures the amplitude of the eye's side-to-side excursion and the total duration in seconds of ocular movements following 10 rotations to the left and 10 rotations to the right while sitting on a manually rotated board.[1] After the SCPNT was published, researchers used it to study postrotary nystagmus in children with learning disabilities,[2-6] hyperactivity,[7] autism,[8-9] behavioral disorders,[10] communicative disorders,[11] and mental retardation.[12] As the use of Ayres' postrotary nystagmus test increased, questions about reliability and clinical significance arose. The purpose of this paper is to review and evaluate the literature which has addressed these issues.

RELIABILITY

The reliability of both excursion and duration of postrotary nystagmus has been studied using the SCPNT. Researchers have examined inter-rater reliability, test-retest reliability, and correlations between visual

Rebecca E. Dutton is Assistant Professor of Occupational Therapy, School of Allied Health Professions, Department of Occupational Therapy, Louisiana State University Medical Center, 1900 Gravier Street, New Orleans, LA 70112-2988.

estimates and electronystagmography (ENG) recordings of postrotary nystagmus. A few investigators have also compared rotary to caloric nystagmus.

Excursion

The reliability of the examiner's visual estimate of the size of the eye's side-to-side excursion during postrotary nystagmus has been investigated. In two studies the test-retest reliability coefficients were .48[1] and .69.[13] Inter-rater reliability for excursion was described as "low" in a third study.[14] Keating showed that the correlation between visual estimates of excursion and ENG recordings of excursion was .61 for normal adults and insignificant for normal children.[15] These data suggest that the use of visual estimates of excursion is questionable because of low inter-rater reliability, low test-retest reliability, and poor correlations with ENG in normal children.

Duration

Reliability data on duration of postrotary nystagmus, on the other hand, are reassuring. Inter-rater reliability coefficients for visual observation of total duration ranged from .97 to .99 in normal and abnormal infants and children.[12,14,16] Test-retest reliability coefficients ranged from .79 to .81 for normal 4 to 11-year-old children.[1,13,17-19] Deitz and associates, however, found lower test-retest correlations for 3-year-old children (.57 for boys and .76 for girls).[17] This may be related to the finding that only 54 percent of the normal 3-year-old children were able to maintain 30 degrees of neck flexion during rotation and only 46 percent were able to maintain their sitting balance when rotation stopped. Without special equipment or modifications the SCPNT requires postural stability which may be beyond some normal 3-year-old capabilities.

Tibbling stated that the duration of rotary-induced nystagmus is a poor measure to use with children. He was specifically referring to normal 3 to 12-month-old infants who have a significantly shorter duration of per-rotary nystagmus, which is offset by a greater speed of eye movements, as compared to normal 1 to 15-year-old children.[20] He thinks that the use of duration scores alone does not allow the examiner to appreciate fully the infant's overall "strength of vestibular activity."[20(p465)] Since additional methods of assessing the vestibular system are available, such as evaluating balance reactions and muscle tone (see previous article in this issue) the use of duration without knowing the speed of nystagmus in infants does not seem as crucial for occupational therapists. Therapists should be aware, however, that duration is significantly shorter for infants than for children, at least as far as the per-rotary procedure is concerned.

Keating studied the accuracy of assessing duration using visual observation versus ENG recordings.[15] She found a correlation of .90 for 20 normal adults and .95 for 4 normal children. A correlation of .63 was found between visually and ENG obtained scores in 4 learning disabled children but it was not statistically significant. Scores differed by a mean of 1.6 seconds in learning disabled subjects with 1mm or more of excursion. Only in subjects with excursions of less than 1mm did the 2 types of scores differ by a mean of 5 seconds. Additional research using a larger sample of learning disabled children is needed to confirm whether children with small eye excursions are the more difficult to measure reliably with visual observation skills. For normal subjects, however, no significant measurement error occurs when assessing duration by visual observation.

The reliability of postrotary nystagmus duration obtained by the SCPNT is excellent as seen by high inter-rater reliability, by strong correlations between ENG recordings and visual observation in normal subjects, and by good test-retest reliability in normal 4 to 11-year-old children.

Caloric Versus Rotary Nystagmus

Some controversy exists over the lack of correlation between caloric and rotary nystagmus testing. Eviatar evaluated 677 children and adults who had vertigo by using both caloric and per-rotary procedures.[21] Caloric nystagmus was induced by placing warm and then cold water in each ear. Per-rotary nystagmus was produced by rotating the subject very slowly so that nystagmus could be recorded during rather than after rotation as in the postrotary procedure. Agreement concerning the presence or absence of nystagmus occurred in 660 of the 677 cases, however, disagreement was present in 61.1 percent of Eviatar's cases when comparing directional and labyrinthine preponderance. This comparison involved counting the number of beats or measuring the speed of eye movements to the left and to the right. When a greater number of beats or faster eye movements occur in one direction versus the other, a preponderance is said to exist. The lack of agreement between caloric and rotary procedures in Eviatar's study was related to preponderance issues, but not to the presence or absence of nystagmus.

A more relevant issue to users of the SCPNT is the reliability of duration during caloric versus rotary nystagmus. Eviatar and Eviatar found that the duration of caloric nystagmus was highly variable in normal children ages birth to 4 years.[22] They felt the repeated positional changes and repeated irrigation of each ear required by the standard caloric procedure contributed to this variability. Baloh and others also found high variability in duration scores during caloric procedures.[23] In fact they found the variability of duration during caloric stimulation was double the variability

of duration following rotary stimulation. Except for cases of partial unilateral peripheral vestibular lesions which frequently go undetected with
rotary testing, Baloh and associates recommended rotary over caloric
testing because of its smaller variability.

VARIABILITY IN ABNORMAL CHILDREN

The duration of postrotary nystagmus in normal adults and children is
reliable as seen by high inter-rater and test-retest reliability as well as
strong correlations between visual observation and ENG recordings. Yet,
no significant correlation was found between visual and ENG findings
with four learning disabled children.[15] The results of two studies suggest
that wide fluctuations of duration is an inherent characteristic of some abnormal children. Nelson and associates found that when autistic children
were tested 18 times over a 25 day period, duration scores fluctuated between 0 and 10 seconds for 4 subjects and between 5 and 15 seconds for 3
subjects.[8] Morrison and Sublett[4] found that when 89 learning disabled
children were tested on 2 different occasions, the children had significantly greater variability in duration than did a normative sample. Forty-five
percent of the children with total duration of 14 seconds or less had scores
which changed by more than one standard deviation at the second test administration. Factors which may be producing this variability include
arousal, visual fixation, and head position.

Arousal

The high variability of nystagmus duration in abnormal children may
be related to variability in arousal level. The results of two studies suggest
that the duration of postrotary nystagmus changes significantly with
changes in arousal level prior to testing.[24,25] When subjects were less alert
they had significantly shorter duration of nystagmus. Pendelton and
Paine[26] found that premature infants, who were more difficult to arouse
fully than full-term infants, initially had shorter duration scores, however, when the premature infants were thoroughly alert, they demonstrated duration scores which were similar to those of full-term infants.
Research on cats suggests this link between arousal and nystagmus may
be found in the reticular formation.[27] When drugs were used that suppress
the reticular formation or when surgical ablations of the reticular formation were performed, the quick component of nystagmus was depressed.
These fast, compensatory eye movements are the reticular formation's attempt to return the eyes to midline with the result being an overshooting
movement toward the direction of rotation.[28] The fluctuations in nystagmus duration in abnormal children may be the result of fluctuations in

the arousal level of the reticular formation and its effect on the quick phase of nystagmus rather than daily changes in the vestibular system or poor test reliability. Morrison and Sublett[4] suggest that therapists obtain a range of scores based on repeated testing to evaluate nystagmus to allow for the possibility of greater day-to-day variability in abnormal children.

Visual Fixation

Visual fixation on a stationary object following rotation has also been explored as a possible factor which affects the reliability of postrotary nystagmus.[29-31] Ornitz and others conducted a definitive study on six different visual fixation conditions.[31] In the two conditions which are relevant to Ayres' test procedure, they compared postrotary nystagmus in a lighted room versus a lighted room with a fixation object present. Duration of postrotary nystagmus did not differ significantly in these two conditions.

Head Position

The inability to hold the head in midline during rotation affected the duration of postrotary nystagmus in Fukuda's study of 70 normal adults.[32] When the subject's head deviated towards the direction of rotation, the mean number of eye beats in 21 seconds decreased. When the subject's head deviated away from the direction of rotation, the number of beats increased. This issue is particularly relevant to abnormal children who exhibit poor postural stability during rotation.[1,11,12] Whether these changes in the number of beats of postrotary nystagmus resulting from head deviation to left or right are statistically significant or would affect duration scores needs further investigation.

CLINICAL SIGNIFICANCE

Once a therapist obtains a raw score on the SCPNT and converts it into a standard deviation score, the process of interpretation can begin. A test must not only be reliable, but the conclusions we draw about a test score must be valid. Researchers have investigated normative guidelines, the clinical significance of prolonged versus depressed nystagmus, and the absence of nystagmus in high-risk infants.

Normative Guidelines

In her normative study, Ayres showed that no significant changes in the duration of postrotary nystagmus occur with increasing age in normal 5 to 9 year old children.[1] Using additional normative samples Punwar[13] and Kimball[33] concurred with this finding. The sex differences in Ayres' normative study[1] were not consistently substantiated by later research. Crowe and associates[34] and Punwar[13] showed that boys' duration scores were significantly longer than those of girls. In several other studies, however, investigators found that sex differences did not reach statistical significance.[19,33,35]

Kimball found a significantly larger standard deviation in normal children than did Ayres.[33] Others[12,17,33-36] have indicated that samples of normal 4 to 9 year old children may have single standard deviation scores ($\pm$ 1.0) which range from a total duration of 6.4 to 32.0 seconds. This raw score range is in excess of 1 standard deviation on the SCPNT which only ranged from 11.7 to 27.3 seconds. Ayres suggested in her test manual that standard deviation scores of -2.0 to $+1.5$ be used as cut-off scores on the postrotary nystagmus test.[1] This would allow children with raw scores from 6 up to 31 seconds to be within normal limits on the test and closely parallels the range of 6 to 32 seconds for normal performance ($\pm$ 1.0 S.D.) established by researchers 5 to 8 years after Ayres' test was published.

Prolonged Nystagmus

Learning disabled children with prolonged duration of postrotary nystagmus have demonstrated deficits in visual perception, spatial relations, and poor paper and pencil skills, such as design copying.[2,3,6,37,38] Eviatar and Eviatar believe that these perceptual-motor deficits are associated with a central rather than a peripheral vestibular problem.[37] Ayres[3] has speculated that damage may occur which affects both "visual-space perception" and higher centers which usually inhibit the vestibular nucleii. All of Ayres' subjects with prolonged nystagmus had "extensive neurological damage" and some even had noticeable left hemisphere damage.[3] Frank and Levison also found that 97 percent of 115 dyslexic children had cerebellar-vestibular dysfunction.[39] They stated that the "cerebellar vestibular system provides the essential background needed for visual perception by means of automatic, integrated motor activity of the eye muscles, head, and neck".[39(p696)] Current research suggests that prolonged postrotary nystagmus is often associated with more extensive damage which affects both cortical and sub-cortical functions. Whether these functions are impaired by a single lesion or a series of lesions is still unknown.

Depressed Nystagmus

Learning disabled children with depressed duration of postrotary nystagmus have consistently demonstrated deficits in muscle tone, balance, and postural control.[2,5,37,40-42] This is not surprising since the vestibular system's primary responsibility is to oppose gravity and initiate balance reactions.[28] Short and associates found that 50 percent of the variance in the duration of postrotary nystagmus in normal pre-school children with depressed nystagmus was accounted for by a cluster of eight variables including prone extension posture, elbow hyperextension, and static standing balance among others.[35] Conversely, Ottenbacher reported that 61 percent of the variance in upper extremity muscle tone was accounted for by prone extension, cocontraction, and postrotary nystagmus.[5] While static standing balance was not a significant predictor of nystagmus duration in Clyse and Short's study, dynamic standing balance did account for 33 percent of the variance in their nystagmus duration scores.[42] Bundy and Fisher pointed out that this relationship between depressed nystagmus, muscle tone, and balance is not obligatory.[40] For example, 35 percent of their subjects with good prone extension had abnormal nystagmus duration and 30 percent with poor or absent prone extension had normal nystagmus duration. These findings suggest that clinicians should not use nystagmus as an isolated measure of vestibular related dysfunction and also emphasize the need for further research concerning the validity of postrotary nystagmus as a measure of vestibular function.

More recently Ayres found that depressed postrotary nystagmus is associated with delayed auditory-language skill.[3] In one sample of learning disabled children 55 percent of the subjects with depressed nystagmus also had an auditory-language deficit. She pointed out that whether this association is a causal relationship is still not known.

Infants

As interest in the vestibular system has grown, occupational therapists have begun to assess postrotary nystagmus in infants. The studies on nystagmus in infants actually pre-dated Ayres' 1975 normative study. In 1973 Brazelton[43] described a "tonic deviation of head and eyes" procedure to test nystagmus which was originally called the "Rotation Test" by Prechtl and Beintema.[44] Brazelton implied, and Prechtl and Beintema stated that the absence of nystagmus in neonates indicated disturbed vestibular function. Yet Mitchell and Cambon[45] found that, at two weeks of age, only 58 percent of normal infants had postrotary nystagmus. Rossi and colleagues found that even at 45 weeks of age, only 83 percent of normal infants had postrotary nystagmus.[46] They also found that a statistically significant increase in the number of normal infants who exhibited nystagmus occurred between the thirty-eighth and forty-second week of life. The absence, therefore, of postrotary nystagmus in infants, particularly those who are under 8 months of age, is not necessarily unusual.

Studies of high-risk infants show that early delays in postrotary nystagmus are not necessarily permanent. Several researchers found that 90 to

100 percent of premature and small-for-gestational age infants developed rotary-induced nystagmus by 12 months of age.[21,46,47]

DeGangi, however, found that 31 of 55 high-risk infants ages 3 to 24 months had abnormal durations of postrotary nystagmus.[14] Twenty-five of these 31 infants had abnormal neurological findings or moderate to severe motor delays on the Bayley motor scale, or both. Earlier researchers were careful to screen out infants with abnormal neonatal courses which may explain the disparity of their findings from those of DeGangi. In the absence of abnormal neurological signs or delayed motor development, high-risk infants under 12 months of age with delayed onset of nystagmus can have a positive outcome. The isolated absence of postrotary nystagmus in such high-risk infants should not necessarily be a cause for alarm. At this age repeated screening of postrotary nystagmus would appear to be more appropriate than early intervention when no other problems exist.

CONCLUSIONS

The purpose of this paper was to examine the reliability of the *Southern California Postrotary Nystagmus Test* and the validity of clinical conclusions which are based on this test. This instrument does have adequate reliability for total duration scores in normal 4 to 11-year-old children as seen by high inter-rater and test-retest reliability coefficients and strong correlations between ENG recordings and visual observations of postrotary nystagmus duration. Physical modification of the nystagmus board for use with children who are under 4 years of age is recommended. Some younger children may not have the postural stability needed for this test which could affect the test-retest reliability of their test scores. The use of eye excursions is not recommended because of its low reliability.

Despite high test reliability in normal subjects, test scores of abnormal subjects often show considerable variance. Research suggests that this variability is an inherent characteristic of some abnormal populations such as autistic or learning disabled children.

Research has demonstrated that nystagmus duration can be significantly affected by arousal level. As arousal increases or decreases, postrotary nystagmus duration increases or decreases respectively. The fluctuations we see in abnormal childrens' postrotary nystagmus may be related to fluctuations in the arousal level of the reticular formation rather than daily changes in the vestibular system. For this reason, researchers recommend that therapists perform repeated testing to obtain a range of scores for abnormal children, particularly for children with a total duration of 14 seconds or less.

Additional normative studies have confirmed the lack of change in duration with increasing age in 4 to 11 year old children. The sex differences found in Ayres' original sample have not been consistently substantiated. Although boys frequently have a larger raw score than girls, this difference was not statistically significant in many of the reviewed studies. These later normative studies have, however, confirmed Ayres' recommendation that standard deviation scores of -2.0 to $+1.5$ on her test should be considered within normal limits. Several studies show that normal 4 to 9-year-old children can exhibit 1 standard deviation around the mean which ranges from 6 to 32 seconds.

Learning disabled children with prolonged postrotary nystagmus duration scores tend to have poor visual perception and poor paper and pencil skills, whereas those with depressed duration tend to have auditory-language deficits. Yet, in some children, delayed visual skills are not paired with prolonged nystagmus and delayed language skills are not associated with depressed nystagmus. Why some children have these clusters of delayed skills and others do not is not known. Similarly, many, but not all, learning disabled children with depressed duration of postrotary nystagmus also have poor balance or poor muscle tone. Yet, so many factors can affect nystagmus that clinicians cannot conclude that a vestibular related deficit exists without assessing several measures of balance and muscle tone in addition to postrotary nystagmus testing.

The research with high-risk infants reiterates the need for caution when assessing postrotary nystagmus in isolation. Many high-risk infants who initially have delayed onset of nystagmus finally develop normal nystagmus by 12 months of age. Clinicians particularly need to be conservative when evaluating postrotary nystagmus in infants under 8 months of age because a significant number of normal infants do not develop nystagmus until then. Depressed or absent postrotary nystagmus in infants is a much more valid cause for concern when it appears in conjunction with abnormal neurological findings or delayed motor development than when it is an isolated finding.

A great deal of the data in this literature review were generated by occupational and physical therapists. The SCPNT has stimulated therapists to produce a large and expanding body of research. Additional studies need to be conducted with disordered populations, but with proper precautions regarding the use of isolated postrotary nystagmus scores and more conservative interpretive guidelines, therapists can use the SCPNT with a fair degree of clinical confidence.

REFERENCES

1. Ayres AJ: *Southern California Postrotary Nystagmus Test: Manual.* Los Angeles, Western Psychological Services, 1975.

2. Ayres AJ: *Interpreting the Southern California Postrotary Sensory Integrative Tests.* Los Angeles, Western Psychological Services, 1976.

3. Ayres AJ: Learning disabilities and the vestibular system. *J Learn Disabil* 11(1): 30-41, 1978.

4. Morrison D, Sublett J: Reliability of the Southern California Postrotary Nystagmus Test with learning disabled children. *Am J Occup Ther* 37(10): 694-698, 1983.

5. Ottenbacher K: Identifying vestibular processing dysfunction in learning disabled children. *Am J Occup Ther* 32(4): 217-221, 1978.

6. Ottenbacher K: Excessive postrotary nystagmus duration in learning disabled children. *Am J Occup Ther* 34(1): 40-44, 1980.

7. Steinberg M, Rendle-Short J: Vestibular dysfunction in young children with minor neurological impairment. *Dev Med Child Neurol* 19: 639-651, 1977.

8. Nelson D, Nitzberg L, Hollander T: Visually monitored postrotary nystagmus in seven autistic children. *Am J Occup Ther* 34(6):382-385, 1980.

9. Ritvo, ER, Ornitz EM, Eviatar A, et al.: Depressed postrotary nystagmus in early infantile autism. *Neurology* 19:653-658, 1969.

10. Ottenbacher K, Watson PJ, Short MA: Association between nystagmus hyporeactivity and behavioral problems in learning disabled children. *Am J Occup Ther* 33(5): 317-322, 1979.

11. Stilwell JM, Crowe TK, McCallum LU: Postrotary nystagmus duration as a function of communication disorders. *Am J Occup Ther* 32(4):222-228, 1978.

12. Siegner CB, Crowe TK, Deitz JC: Interrater reliability of the Southern California Postrotary Nystagmus Test. *Phys Occup Ther Pediatr* 2(2/3):83-91, 1982.

13. Punwar A: Expanded normative data: The Southern California Postrotary Nystagmus Test. *Am J Occup Ther* 36(3): 183-187, 1982.

14. DeGangi GA: The relationship of vestibular responses to developmental functions in high risk infants. *Phys Occup Ther Pediatr* 2(2/3):35-49, 1982.

15. Keating NR: A comparison of duration of nystagmus as measured by the SCPNT and electronystagmography. *Am J Occup Ther* 33(2):92-97, 1979.

16. Montgomery P, Rodel D: Effect of state on nystagmus duration on the Southern California Postrotary Nystagmus Test. *Am J Occup Ther* 32(3):177-182, 1982.

17. Deitz J, Seigner C, Crowe T: The Southern California Postrotary Nystagmus Test: Test-retest reliability for pre-school children. *Occup Ther J Res* 1:165-177, 1981.

18. Kimball JG: The Southern California Postrotary Nystagmus Test: Stability over time, in Tyler N (ed): *Integration Topics: Faculty Reviews.* Los Angeles, CSSID Publications, 1980.

19. Royeen CB: Factors affecting test-retest reliability of the Southern California Postrotary Nystagmus Test. *Am J Occup Ther* 34(1):37-39, 1980.

20. Tibbling L: The rotary nystagmus response in children. *Acta Otolaryngol* 68:459-467, 1969.

21. Eviatar A: The torsion swing as a vestibular test. *Arch Otolaryngol* 92:437-444, 1970.

22. Eviatar L, Eviatar A: The normal nystagmic response of infants to caloric and per-rotary stimulation. *Laryngoscope* 89(7): 1036-1044, 1979.

23. Baloh RW, Sills AW, Honrubia V: Impulsive and sinusoidal rotary testing. A comparison with results of caloric testing. *Laryngoscope* 89:646-654, 1979.

24. Montgomery PC, Capps MJ: The effect of arousal on the nystagmus response of normal children. *Phys Occup Ther Pediatr* 1(2):17-29, 1980.

25. Collins WE: The effects of mental set upon vestibular nystagmus. *J Exper Psychol* 63:191-197, 1962.

26. Pendleton M, Paine R: Vestibular nystagmus in newborn infants. *Neurology* 11:450-458, 1961.

27. McCabe BF: The quick component of nystagmus. *Laryngoscope* 75:1619-1646, 1965.

28. Baloh RW, Honrubia V: *Clinical Neurophysiology of the Vestibular System.* Philadelphia, PA Davis Co, 1979.

29. Levy DL, Proctor LR, Holaman PS: Visual interference in the vestibular response. *Arch Otolaryngol* 103:287-291, 1977.

30. Tjernstrom O: Nystagmus inhibition as an effect of eye closure. *Acta Otolaryngol* 75:408-418, 1973.

31. Ornitz EJ, Brown MB, Mason A et al.: The effect of visual input on postrotary nystagmus in normal children. *Acta Otolaryngol* 77:418-425, 1974.

32. Fukuda T: Postural behavior and motion sickness. *Acta Otolaryngol* 81:237-241, 1976.

33. Kimball JG: Normative comparison of the Southern California Postrotary Nystagmus Test: Los Angeles vs Syracuse data. *Am J Occup Ther* 35(1):21-25, 1981.

34. Crowe TK, Deitz JC, Siegner CB: Postrotary nystagmus response of normal four-year-old children. *Phys Occup Ther Pediatr* 4(2):19-28, 1984.

35. Short MA, Watson PJ, Ottenbacher K, et al.: Vestibular-proprioceptive function in four year olds: Normative and regression analysis. *Am J Occup Ther* 37(2):102-109, 1983.

36. Dunn W: *A Guide to Testing Clinical Observations in Kindergartners.* Washington, DC, American Occupational Therapy Association, 1981.

37. Eviatar L, Eviatar A: Neurovestibular examination in infants and children. Read before Third Annual Sensory Integration Symposium, Seattle, WA, June 26-27, 1982.

38. Ottenbacher K: Excessive postrotary nystagmus duration in learning disabled children. *Am J Occup Ther* 34(1):40-44, 1980.

39. Frank J, Levinson H: Dysmetric dyslexia and dyspraxia: Hypothesis and study. *J Amer Acad Child Psychiatry* 12:690-701, 1973.

40. Bundy AC, Fisher AG: The relationship of prone extension to other vestibular functions. *Am J Occup Ther* 35(12):782-787, 1981.

41. DeQuiros JB: Diagnosis of vestibular disorders in the learning disabled. *J Learn Disabil* 9: 50-58, 1976.

42. Clyse SJ, Short MA: The relationship between dynamic balance and postrotary nystagmus in learning disabled children. *Phys Occup Ther Pediatr* 3(3):25-32, 1983.

43. Brazelton TB: *Neonatal Behavioral Assessment Scale.* Clinics in Developmental Medicine, No. 50. Philadelphia, JB Lippincott Co, 1973.

44. Prechtl H, Beintema D: *The Neurological Examination of the Full-term Newborn Infant.* Clinics in Developmental Medicine, No. 12. Philadelphia, JB Lippincott Co, 1964.

45. Mitchell T, Cambon K: Vestibular responses in neonates and infants. *Arch Otolaryngol* 90: 556-557, 1969.

46. Rossi L, Rignataro O, Nino L: Maturation of the vestibular response: A preliminary report. *Dev Med Child Neurol* 21:217-224, 1979.

47. Eviatar L, Eviatar A, Naray I: Maturation of the neurovestibular responses in infants. *Dev Med Child Neurol* 16:435-446, 1974.

Developmental Status of Children Exhibiting Postrotatory Nystagmus Durations of Zero Seconds

Jean C. Deitz, PhD, OTR
Terry K. Crowe, MS, OTR

ABSTRACT. This research, using a sample of 4 1/2 year-old children identified during the first weeks of life as high risk, had two purposes. The first was to describe the developmental status of those children having Southern California Postrotary Nystagmus Test scores of zero seconds. The second was to compare the visual motor, gross motor, and cognitive development of the children with postrotatory nystagmus scores of zero seconds with children having nystagmus durations within a normal range. On all seven measures used in this research, the zero nystagmus group performed worse than the normal nystagmus group. On two measures, the Peabody Developmental Gross Motor Scale and scissor cutting errors, results were significant at p < .007. For three other measures, WPPSI-Verbal, standing balance, and the Frostig Eye-Motor Coordination Subtest, results were significant at p < .05. Possible functional implications for children with zero nystagmus were discussed.

INTRODUCTION

The Southern California Postrotary Nystagmus Test (SCPNT)[1] has been used by therapists in clinical settings for over ten years. Ayres described the SCPNT as one of the better, simple tools to measure the efficiency or integrity of the vestibular system.[2] Expanded normative data have allowed therapists to administer the SCPNT to children covering a wide age span.[3-5] In addition, several reliability and validity studies have been conducted on the SCPNT.[6-10]

Jean C. Deitz is an occupational therapy assistant professor in the Department of Rehabilitation Medicine, University of Washington, Seattle, WA.

Terry K. Crowe is the head of Occupational Therapy at the Child Development and Mental Retardation Center and an Occupational Therapy faculty member in the Department of Rehabilitation Medicine, University of Washington, Seattle, WA.

The authors express appreciation to Kathy Stewart and Cary Siegner for assisting in data collection, to consultants in the Department of Biostatistics and Charles A. Lund for statistical consultation, to Norma Dermond for data processing, and to the children and their parents for participating in this study.

Depressed postrotatory nystagmus duration, that is nystagmus lower than one standard deviation below the mean, is considered by Ayres to reflect a vestibular processing deficit.[1] Children with depressed nystagmus often have other dysfunctional areas including hypotonicity, motor incoordination, and poor postural and ocular reactions.[10-12] In addition, several researchers suggest that children with short nystagmus durations appear to exhibit problems in visual motor control.[13-15]

While the phenomenon of depressed nystagmus has been well documented in the literature, no one has comprehensively examined a substantial group of children with absolutely no observed postrotatory nystagmus following rotation to both the right and left. Ayres'[1] original standardization sample of 226 children, ages 5 to 9 years, contained no children with nystagmus durations of zero seconds. Four children (6%) in Ayres' sample of 68 learning disabled children, however, had zero seconds of nystagmus following rotation in either direction. It was impossible to determine if any of the children had zero seconds of nystagmus after rotation in both directions. Crowe, Deitz and Siegner[5] found that none of 41 normal 4-year-old children had total nystagmus duration scores of less than four seconds. In contrast, Short and associates found, in a sample of 156 Head Start 4-year-old children, that 7% (7 males, 4 females) exhibited nystagmus durations of zero seconds.[16] This study sample represented a lower class, mixed race, Southern, combined urban and rural population. Kimball,[9] in a normative study, described one well coordinated and academically superior 8-year-old child with no observed postrotatory nystagmus after rotation in both directions. Other normative studies have been conducted but, because of the way the data were reported, whether the samples included children with zero seconds of postrotatory nystagmus could not be determined.

While total nystagmus durations of zero seconds appear to be a relatively rare observation in normal children, therapists testing a group of "high-risk" preschoolers noted a comparatively high incidence of children with zero second SCPNT scores. These subjects were participating in a longitudinal follow-up study of children who were cared for in a Neonatal Intensive Care Unit (NICU) during the first few weeks of life. In view of this observation, this retrospective study was planned with two purposes. The first was to describe the developmental status of 4 1/2-year-old children having SCPNT total scores of zero seconds. The second was to compare the visual motor, gross motor, and cognitive development of the children having SCPNT total scores of zero seconds with those having SCPNT total scores within a normal range. Based on the literature review, we hypothesized that children with zero nystagmus would earn lower scores than children with normal nystagmus on measures of gross motor, balance, visual motor, and prone extension activities. No difference was expected on verbal or performance intelligence. Thus, the following null hypothesis was tested.

No significant difference exists between the scores on developmental assessments earned by children with SCPNT total scores of zero seconds and the scores earned by children with normal SCPNT scores.

This was tested for seven variables: Wechsler Preschool and Primary Scale of Intelligence-Verbal (WPPSI-Verbal), WPPSI—Performance, Peabody Developmental Gross Motor Scale, standing balance-eyes open, Eye-Motor Coordination Subtest of the Frostig Developmental Test of Visual Perception, scissor cutting errors, and modified prone extension.

METHOD

Subjects

As part of the routine follow-up for high risk infants at the University of Washington these children, when they reach an approximate corrected age of 4 1/2 years, are evaluated in occupational therapy and psychology. Ninety-five children (46 males and 49 females) were evaluated between December 1980 and May 1984 who had SCPNT scores, data for all seven variables, and a corrected age between 52 and 56 months at the time of testing. In order to be included in this longitudinal follow-up program these children had to be survivors of idiopathic respiratory distress syndrome, or had to have weighed 1500 grams or less at birth, or had to have had a central nervous system infection or disorder such as meningitis during the first months of life.

For the purposes of this study two groups were identified from this larger group of children. The first group was composed of those children having SCPNT total scores of zero seconds. The second group was composed of those children having normal nystagmus which was defined as having SCPNT total scores within plus or minus one standard deviation of the mean for 4-year-old children.[5] Means and standard deviations used in identifying this group were sex specific.

The zero nystagmus group was comprised of 11 subjects including eight males and three females. All subjects were Caucasian. The normal nystagmus group was composed of 49 subjects including 29 females and 20 males. Of this group 47 subjects were Caucasian and two subjects were Black. Additional characteristics of subjects in each group are reported in Table 1. Thirty-five subjects had nystagmus scores that were not equal to zero but were beyond plus or minus one standard deviation from the mean. These subjects were not included in this study.

Procedure and Instrumentation

For the purposes of this study, scores for each child from the SCPNT and seven other measures were used. The SCPNT and the visual motor and gross motor measures were administered by three registered occupational therapists all of whom have had extensive pediatric experience and are certified to administer the Southern California Postrotary Nystagmus Test.

Using the administration procedure outlined by Crowe, Deitz and Siegner,[5] the SCPNT was administered following sedentary activity. Two measures of visual-motor ability were used. The first was the Eye-Motor

Table 1

Characteristics of Subjects

	N	Mean	Median	SD	High Score-Low-Score
Birthweight (Grams)					
Zero Nystagmus Group	11	1678	1360	847	780-3400
Normal Nystagmus Group	49	1717	1452	878	750-5130
Gestational Age (weeks)					
Zero Nystagmus Group	11	31.7	31.0	4.8	25-41
Normal Nystagmus Group	49	32.5	32.2	3.4	24-40
1-Minute Apgar					
Zero Nystagmus Group	10*	4.1	4.5	2.3	1-7
Normal Nystagmus Group	47**	5.2	5.4	2.5	0-9
5-Minute Apgar					
Zero Nystagmus Group	10*	7.6	7.5	1.4	6-9
Normal Nystagmus Group	43**	7.4	7.9	1.9	2-10

*   Agpar scores were missing for one subject because of a precipitous home delivery.

**   Agpar scores were missing from medical charts either because of complications during and/or shortly after delivery or for unspecified reasons.

Coordination Subtest of the Frostig Developmental Test of Visual Perception.[17] The test items require the child to draw straight or curved lines between progressively narrower boundaries and to draw straight lines to a target. Interrater reliability data were available only for test administrators one and three for a sample of 10 children (r = .93). The second measure of visual motor ability, scissor cutting errors, was adapted from the research edition of the Miller Assessment for Preschoolers.[18] After the child practiced cutting along a 12-inch straight line that was one-eighth inch thick, the child was asked to cut around a 4-inch circle that was three-sixteenths of an inch thick. Using a plastic overlay for scoring the circle, the errors (maximum of 48) were counted and recorded. Again, interrater reliability data were available only for test administrators one and three (r = .79). This was calculated for a sample of 8 children.

As a comprehensive measure of gross motor ability, the Peabody Developmental Gross Motor Scale (one of two scales in the Peabody Developmental Motor Scales—revised experimental edition) was administered.[19] This scale includes items involving balance, ball handling skill, and developmental motor milestones such as running, hopping, skipping, and jumping. Interrater reliabilities were high for the measure (r = .99 for test administrators one and two using a sample of 10 children; r = .98 for test administrators one and three using a sample of 8 children). A standing balance item from this measure also was used as an isolated variable. This item required that the child stand on one foot with hands on hips and eyes open. The child was timed to see how long this posture could be maintained without putting the raised foot on the floor, without changing upper extremity position, and without hopping or otherwise moving the weight-bearing foot. This was then repeated for the opposite leg. Two trials were given for each leg and the longest duration for each leg was used in computing a total score. A maximum possible total score was set at 30 seconds. The last motor measure was the modified prone extension posture, whereby the children were positioned in prone and asked to lift their heads, trunks, and extremities off the surface. Lower extremity extension was omitted. The child's performance on this measure was graded on a 6-point scale based on the length of time the child maintained the required posture (1 = 0 seconds, 2 = 1-5 seconds, 3 = 6-10 seconds, 4 = 11-15 seconds, 5 = 16-20 seconds, 6 = 21 or more seconds). Interrater reliability studies for this measure indicated that the examiners were highly reliable in their ratings (r = 1.00 for test administrators one and two using a sample of 5 children; r = .98 for test administrators one and three using a sample of 8 children.

The Wechsler Preschool and Primary Scales of Intelligence[20] were used as measures of cognitive ability. These were administered by a variety of psychologists and no interrater reliability data were available.

Research and Statistical Design

This was a retrospective study whereby the performance of two groups on seven variables were described and compared. Since data from modified prone extension were ordinal, data for the two groups were to be compared using a Mann-Whitney *U*. For all other variables, *t*-test comparisons were to be made unless the assumptions for use of this statistic were not met, thus requiring the use of non-parametric statistics. Because we hypothesized that the normal nystagmus group would perform significantly better than the zero nystagmus group on measures of gross motor, balance, visual motor and modified prone extension, one-tailed tests of probability were employed for comparisons involving these measures. Two-tailed tests of probability were used for WPPSI-Verbal and WPPSI-Performance since the direction of the difference was not hypothesized for these variables.

Because this was an exploratory study and the sample size was small, thus limiting power, the decision was made to set alpha at .05. Since multiple comparisons were to be made, the likelihood of making a type I error was increased and thus findings at or near this level should be viewed with caution and as a guide for future research. In order to correct for the use of seven statistical tests a second alpha was set at .007 for each separate test. This was done using the least significant difference (LSD) method[21] whereby the significance level of each separate test is set at the desired overall significance level (p = .05) divided by the number of separate comparisons (7). We reasoned that if any variables met the standards for this very conservative method of adjustment, one could have reasonable confidence in those findings.

RESULTS

Data describing the motor and cognitive performance of the children in this study with zero nystagmus and that of the children in this study with normal nystagmus appear in Table 2. On all measures except scissor cutting errors, higher scores were indicative of higher levels of function. As can be noted, the normal nystagmus group received better scores on all measures than the zero nystagmus group.

The zero nystagmus group and the normal nystagmus group were compared on seven variables. Visual inspection of the data and initial analyses using the Kolmogorov-Smirnov two-sample test indicated that the distributions of five of the variables met the assumption of normality. These analyses further indicated that two variables (scissor cutting errors and modified prone extension) did not meet this assumption. Using a base 10 logarithmic transformation,[22] scissor cutting errors met the assumption of

Table 2

Cognitive and Motor Performance of Children with Zero Nystagmus (n=11) and

Children with Normal Nystagmus (n=49)

	Mean	S.D.	Median	Low Score-High Score	T-Value	Two-Tailed Probability	One-Tailed Probability
WPPSI-Verbal							
Zero Nystagmus Children	97.9	16.6	105.0	66-124			
					-2.24	.029	
Normal Nystagmus Children	108.3	13.3	109.8	69-146			
WPPSI-Performance							
Zero Nystagmus Children	102.8	15.1	101.0	81-129			
					-1.55	.127	
Normal Nystagmus Children	109.9	13.4	108.1	82-150			
Peabody Developmental Gross Motor Scale							
Zero Nystagmus Children	131.2	14.8	130.0	113-155			
					-2.67		.005
Normal Nystagmus Children	141.4	10.7	142.8	115-156			
Standing Balance							
Zero Nystagmus Children	10.5	10.0	7.0	1-30			
					-1.96		.028
Normal Nystagmus Children	16.4	8.7	15.3	0-30			
Frostig Eye-Motor Coordination Subtest							
Zero Nystagmus Children	6.6	2.1	6.3	4-11			
					-1.86		.034
Normal Nystagmus Children	8.4	3.1	8.4	3-15			
Scissor Cutting (Number of Errors							
Zero Nystagmus Children	21.9	18.1	12.0	4-43			
					2.76		.004
Normal Nystagmus Children	9.6	11.8	5.8	0-48			

normality, thus making t-test comparisons possible for six variables. Since the assumption of homogeneity of variance was met for these six variables, the pooled variance estimate was used. Results indicated that the normal nystagmus group performed significantly better on five measures (Table 2). On two of these measures, the Peabody Developmental Gross Motor Scale and scissor cutting errors, results were significant beyond the second alpha level of .007 (one-tailed). For two measures, standing balance and the Frostig Eye-Motor Coordination Subtest, results were significant at p < .05 (one-tailed) and for WPPSI-Verbal, results were significant at p < .05 (two-tailed). The null hypothesis was not rejected for WPPSI-Performance.

For the last variable, prone extension, the zero nystagmus group had a median of 5.0 which was slightly lower than the median of 5.6 for the normal nystagmus group. For both groups, prone extension scores ranged from one to six. A Mann-Whitney U test,[23] used to compare the performance of the two groups of this measure, was not significant, corrected $z = 1.30$, p = .096 (one-tailed).

DISCUSSION

The normal nystagmus group performed better than the zero nystagmus group on all seven measures of gross motor, visual motor and cognitive development used in this study. A relatively comprehensive gross motor evaluation, the Peabody Developmental Gross Motor Scale, was used to assess a wide range of motor activities typically engaged in by the young child. As a result, the finding that the zero nystagmus group performed significantly worse, p < .007 (one-tailed), on this measure could have functional implications for the young child with zero nystagmus. It suggests that such children might have difficulties engaging in motor activities common to their age groups.

On the second gross motor measure, standing balance, the performance of the zero nystagmus group was again significantly lower, p < .05 (one-tailed), than the performance of the normal nystagmus group. This finding is in concurrence with the literature on depressed postrotatory nystagmus. Three studies, two with learning disabled children[10,11] and one with Head Start Children,[16] revealed relationships between nystagmus duration scores and measures of standing balance with open eyes.

On the third gross motor measure, modified prone extension, the performance of the zero nystagmus group was lower but not significantly different from that of the normal nystagmus group. This finding was not expected for modified prone extension in view of the literature[10,11,16] suggesting a relationship between this variable and SCPNT. Ayres suggests that inability of a child with minimal brain dysfunction to assume and maintain a prone extension posture can be interpreted as a vestibular processing deficit.[24] Three factors that may have influenced the findings in relationship to prone extension in the current study merit consideration. First, the prone extension measure was the only variable tested with the Mann-Whitney *U*. The lower power of this test may have reduced its ability to detect a statistically significant difference between the two groups. Second, this difference in findings may be the result of modifications in both the prone extension posture and the scoring system in the current study. The modification in the posture was made in view of Harris's findings for children of a preschool age.[25] Third, the prone extension posture, even with modification, may not be a good discriminator among 4-year-old children. When Gregory-Flock and Yerxa[26] compared a small group of learning-disabled children with a nondisabled group, the prone extension postural test did not differentiate between the two groups of 4-year-olds. In all other age groups (5 through 8 years), the normal children scored significantly higher in both duration and quality on the prone extension postural test. Harris[25] concluded that the variability of performance by 4-year-olds indicates that the ability to assume and maintain a prone extension position is not a valid measurement for discriminating between normal children and those "at risk" for learning disabilities at this age level.

In addition to performing worse on a comprehensive measure of gross motor development and a standing balance measure, the zero nystagmus group performed significantly worse than the normal nystagmus group on both measures of visual motor skill, the Frostig Eye-Motor Coordination Subtest, $p < .05$ (one-tailed) and scissor cutting errors, $p < .007$ (one-tailed). This finding parallels several studies in the literature that suggest a linkage between depressed nystagmus and visual motor coordination.[13-15] Again, this finding has functional implications since the visual motor assessments used in the current study required skills (i.e., scissor cutting precision and paper-pencil control) necessary for successfully meeting the demands in the later preschool and grade school environments.

Our findings further suggested that children with normal nystagmus perform better than children with zero nystagmus on verbal intelligence, $p < .05$. This finding again reflects the literature on depressed nystagmus. In a population of 92 learning disabled children, Ayres found that of the 53 percent of those with language disorders, 55 percent exhibited depressed postrotatory nystagmus.[12] Stillwell, Crowe, and McCallum[27] reported that children with communication disorders had significantly depressed mean durations of postrotatory nystagmus compared to a control group of normal children ($p < .05$). The difference between the two groups on WPPSI-Performance was not significant at $p < .05$.

In addition to the findings about specific variables, two general findings were of interest. First, more males than females had zero seconds of postrotatory nystagmus. This was similar to the findings reported by Short and associates.[16] Second, was that, of the ninety-five 4 1/2-year-old children meeting the criteria for inclusion in this study, 11 children (11.6%) had zero nystagmus. This frequency of zero total scores on the SCPNT differs from that found by Crowe, Deitz and Siegner[5] for 41 normal 4-year-old children. In this group none of the children had zero SCPNT total scores or zero scores for either the right or the left. This is particularly noteworthy in view of three considerations. First the children in both studies lived in the same area of the country. Second, the children in both studies were more than 4 years of age but less than 5 years of age. Third, the test administrator for the study with normal children also was one of three therapists involved in evaluating the children identified as high risk. In a previous project she had demonstrated high interrater reliabilities (normal, r = .964; developmentally different, r = .992) for total scores with one of the other test administrators for the NICU Follow-Up project.[7] The third test administrator for this project was certified to administer the SCPNT and was further trained by the other two evaluators. Using a sample of normal children, test administrators one and three established a high level of interrater reliability (r = .973) for total SCPNT scores. In view of this, the differences in the frequency of occurrence of zero nystagmus are not likely to be explained by differences in test administration procedures.

In summary, the zero nystagmus group performed worse than the normal nystagmus group on measures of gross motor, visual motor and cognitive development. For two measures, the Peabody Developmental Gross Motor Scales and scissor cutting errors, the results were more highly significant than for WPPSI-Verbal, standing balance, and the Frostig Eye-Motor Coordination Subtest. The findings for the latter three variables should be viewed with caution because of the borderline probability levels and in view of the multiple comparisons in this study. In addition this sample of high risk children had a higher proportion of children with zero nystagmus than that reported for normal children of the same age[5] and more males than females had zero seconds of postrotatory nystagmus.

REFERENCES

1. Ayres AJ: *Southern California Postrotary Nystagmus Test Manual.* Los Angeles, Western Psychological Services, 1975.

2. Ayres AJ: *Sensory Integration and the Child.* Los Angeles, Western Psychological Services, 1975.

3. Kaufman CJ: Postrotary Nystagmus in Three, Four, and Five Year Old Children. Thesis, Colorado State University, 1978.

4. Punwar A: Expanded normative data: Southern California Postrotary Nystagmus Test. *Am J Occup Ther* 36:183-187, 1982.

5. Crowe TK, Deitz JC, Siegner CB: Postrotatory nystagmus response of normal 4-year-old children. *Phys Occup Ther Pediatr* 4(2):19-28, 1984.

6. Deitz, JC, Siegner CB, Crowe TK: The Southern California Postrotary Nystagmus Test: Test-retest reliability for preschool children. *Occup Ther J Res* 1:165-177, 1981.

7. Siegner CB, Crowe TK, Deitz JC: Interrater reliability of the Southern California Postrotary Nystagmus Test. *Phys Occup Ther Pediatr* 2(2/3):83-91, 1982.

8. Morrison D, Sublett J: Reliability of the Southern California Postrotary Nystagmus Test with learning-disabled children. *Am J Occup Ther* 37:694-698, 1983.

9. Kimball J: Normative comparison of the Southern California Postrotary Nystagmus Test: Los Angeles vs Syracuse Data. *Am J Occup Ther* 35:21-25, 1981.

10. Ottenbacher K: Identifying vestibular processing dysfunction in learning-disabled children. *Am J Occup Th* 32:217-221, 1978.

11. Clyse SJ, Short MA: The relationship between dynamic balance and postrotary nystagmus in learning disabled children. *Phys Occup Ther Pediatr* 3(3):25-31, 1983.

12. Ayres AJ: Learning disabilities and the vestibular system. *J Learn Disabil* 11:30-41, 1978.

13. Watson PJ, Ottenbacher K, Short MA et al.: Human figure drawings of learning disabled children with hyporesponsive postrotary nystagmus. *Phys Occup Ther Pediatr* 1(4):21-25, 1981.

14. Ottenbacher K, Watson PJ, Short MA, Biderman MD: Nystagmus and ocular fixation difficulties in learning-disabled children. *Am J Occup Th* 33:717-721, 1979.

15. Watson PJ, Ottenbacher K, Workmen EA, et al.: Visual motor difficulties in emotionally disturbed children with hyporesponsive nystagmus. *Phys Occup Ther Pediatr* 2(2/3):67-71, 1982.

16. Short MA, Watson PJ, Ottenbacher K, Rogers C: Vestibular proprioceptive functions in 4 year olds: Normative and regression analyses. *Am J Occup Th* 37:102-109, 1983.

17. Frostig M, Maslow P, Lefever DW, Wittlesey JRB: *The Marianne Frostig Developmental Test of Visual Perception—1963 Standardization*. California, Consulting Psychologist Press, 1964.

18. Miller LJ: Personal communication, 1983.

19. Folio R, Dubose RF: Peabody Developmental Motor Scales (revised experimental edition). *IMRID Behavioral Science Monograph No. 25*, 1974.

20. Wechsler D: *Manual for the Wechsler Preschool and Primary Scale of Intelligence*. New York, Psychological Corporation, 1967.

21. Kleinbaum DG, Kuppe LL: *Applied Regression Analysis and Other Multi-variable Methods*. Massachusetts, Duxbury Press, 1978.

22. Nie NH, Hull CH, Jenkins JG et al.: *Statistical Package for the Social Sciences*. New York, McGraw-Hill Book Company, 1975.

23. Siegel S: *Nonparametric Statistics for the Behavioral Sciences*. New York, McGraw-Hill Book Company, 1956.

24. Ayres AJ: *Interpreting the Southern California Sensory Integrations Tests*. Los Angeles, Western Psychological Services, 1976.

25. Harris NP: Duration and quality of the prone extension position in four- six- and eight-year old normal children. *Am J Occup Ther* 35:16-30, 1981.

26. Gregory-Flock J, Yerxa EJ: Standardization of the Prone Extension Postural Test on children ages 4 through 8. *Am J Occup Ther* 38:187-194, 1984.

27. Stillwell JM, Crowe TK, McCallum: Postrotatory nystagmus duration as a function of communication disorder. *Am J Occup Ther* 32:222-228, 1978.

Immediate Effects
of Waterbed Flotation on Approach
and Avoidance Behaviors
of Premature Infants

Judith M. Pelletier, MS, OTR
Margaret A. Short, PhD, OTR
David L. Nelson, PhD, OTR

ABSTRACT. This study was designed to determine the immediate effects of waterbed flotation on approach and avoidance movements in premature infants. Twenty-two premature infants free of major medical complications were randomly assigned to experimental (n = 11) or control (n = 11) groups. After each of five consecutive gavage feedings, each infant in the experimental group was placed for 30 minutes on a Medpro Neo-Float Neonatal Flotation System with oscillating dual frequency rhythmic wave stimulator. Control group infants were placed on standard isolette mattresses. Differences between groups were highly significant on five of six behaviors observed, with the occurrence of hand-to-mouth greater and the frequencies of grimace, startle, trunkal arch, and salute behaviors less in the experimental group than in the control group. No significant differences were noted on finger splaying. These results have possible implications both for the routine use of waterbeds in intensive care nurseries and for the specialized use of waterbeds in infant stimulation programs.

Judith M. Pelletier is currently with the Division of Neonatology, John Dempsy Hospital, University of Connecticut Health Center, Farmington, CT 06032.

Margaret A. Short and David L. Nelson were on the faculty of the Department of Occupational Therapy, Sargent College of Allied Health Professions, Boston University at the time this study was conducted. Dr. Short is currently practicing in Saratoga Springs, NY. Dr. Nelson is in the Department of Occupational Therapy, Western Michigan University, Kalamazoo, MI.

This investigation was supported in part by a training grant from the Bureau of Community Health Services, Maternal and Child Health, Project 906, which was administered through the Eunice Kennedy Shriver Center, Waltham, MA. Thanks are due to Molly Kingsbury, RN for her technical assistance and to Heidelise Als, for consultation in the planning stages of this project. For their support and assistance in carrying out this study, the following are acknowledged: John Raye, Hema DeSilva and the staff of the Neonatal Intensive Care Units of the University of Connecticut Health Center, Farmington, CT and the Saint Francis Hospital and Medical Center, Hartford, CT; Medpro Inc. for supplying waterbed equipment, and Ohio Medical Products for temporary loan of an isolette.

Parts of this manuscript were reported in a presentation to the New England Perinatal Society, Annual Meeting, 1983.

INTRODUCTION

Various types of sensory stimulation have been shown to have positive effects on the behavior and development of premature infants.[1-4] Because it appears and matures early, the vestibular system has been proposed to be one of the most effective vehicles for providing developmentally relevant stimulation to the newborn infant.[5-7] This system is also thought to play a role in motor development and has been explored as a means of influencing the development of premature and term infants.[8,9] In general, vestibular stimulation is claimed to effect behavioral and developmental changes in infants; and the vestibular system is claimed to mediate changes such as more efficient visual pursuit,[10] increased relaxation,[11] calming,[12] the inhibition of crying and the enhancement of visual alertness in infants.[13] Animal studies have also pointed to the possible functional value of vestibular stimulation for survival and development of human neonates.[14-16]

Premature infants, who are deprived of full exposure to the intrauterine environment, have demonstrated responsiveness to extrauterine stimulation. Neal[17] reasoned that, since the vestibular system is one of the first sensory systems to develop, and since premature infants might be deprived of rhythmical vestibular stimulation in utero, premature infants might be more receptive to vestibular than to any other type of sensory stimulation. She demonstrated that a daily regimen of rocking caused significant advances in motor, visual and auditory responses in an experimental group of premature infants. Similarly, Barnard[18] showed that rocking and auditory stimulation caused significantly greater increases in the amount and length of quiet sleep as well as a trend toward greater weight gain and higher maturational scores in an experimental group of premature infants. Rose[19] concluded that, although visual recognition memory is negatively affected by prematurity, it can be improved by altering early environmental conditions with combined tactile, kinesthetic, vestibular and auditory stimulation.

The development of a neonatal waterbed and the use of waterbed flotation in developmental studies began in 1972 as an extension of examinations of the effects of vestibular-proprioceptive stimulation on the development of premature infants. The waterbed is highly responsive to even small movements and is thought to provide tactile-kinesthetic and vestibular-proprioceptive feedback. The waterbed itself provides some containment of the infant via cradling in the slight depression caused by the weight of the infant's body, and gentle oscillations of the waterbed may add further vestibular and possible proprioceptive stimulation. For these reasons, the oscillating waterbed has been seen as a means of simulating aspects of the intrauterine environment while providing vestibular-proprioceptive stimulation without additional handling.[20]

The safety of waterbed use with premature infants was determined by

Korner and associates[7] who demonstrated no change in pulse, respiration, temperature, weight, and oxygen requirement but a significant decrease in apnea with the use of oscillating waterbeds. Korner, Guilleminault, Van den Hoed and Baldwin[21] subsequently conducted a study involving polygraphically recorded sleep and respiratory patterns of premature infants who were preselected for apnea and placed on waterbeds. Their results confirmed that the oscillating waterbed has apnea-reducing effects. This was further supported by Korner, Ruppel and Rho,[22] who examined the effects of waterbeds on the sleep and motility of premature infants treated with theophylline, a drug which reduces apnea but which increases wakefulness and erratic motor behavior. The results of this study indicated that infants had more quiet and active sleep, shorter sleep latencies, fewer state changes, less restlessness during sleep, less waking activity, and fewer jittery and unsmooth movements when on the waterbed than when under the control condition.

Potential clinical benefits derived from the waterbed include decreasing the incidence of the development of asymmetrically shaped heads, decreasing the frequency of intracranial bleeds, and conserving energy by decreasing the full impact of gravity. Additionally, waterbeds are claimed to be useful in the prevention of skin breakdown in small infants, for infants who are recovering from abdominal surgery or who are on parenteral nutrition.[20,23]

In general, waterbeds positively affect the organization of infants' behaviors. For example, the movements of infants on waterbeds appear to be smoother and less random, with fewer overshooting movements and fewer startles than infants on standard mattresses. Infants on waterbeds also seem to be more able to establish hand-to-mouth contact.[20] Kramer and Pierpoint[23] examined the effects of flotation on a gently rocking waterbed combined with auditory stimulation via a taped simulated heart beat and a woman's voice, and reported significant increases in weight, head circumference, and anterior-posterior and biparietal diameter of the heads of treatment infants. In addition, the infants on the waterbeds were informally observed to nipple earlier, to eat better and to be more active than controls. Burns,[24] however, reported that use of the waterbed with auditory stimulation (tape of rhythmic sounds of placental blood flow) increased developmental progress in motor and state organization, while causing no change in daily weight gain, weekly biparietal diameter of the head, or head circumference.

The organization of infant behaviors has been increasingly examined in infant research,[8,25-28] with recent infant assessments including behavioral items[29-31] that reflect the organization of motor behaviors. One model of behavioral organization has been posed in The Assessment of Premature Infant Behavior.[32,33] This model poses that a major task of the developing infant is to gradually coordinate a smooth interaction of two components of behavior, approach and avoidance. A well-regulated balance of these behaviors should allow the infant to participate in adequate adaptive functions.

In light of the previous research regarding the benefits of waterbeds, the present study was designed to test further the effects of waterbeds on adaptive behaviors of premature infants. The infants in this study were all receiving gavage feeding, an invasive procedure which would be expected to disrupt the premature infant's efforts to achieve equilibrium between approach and avoidance behaviors. We hypothesized that, following gavage feeding, infants placed on waterbeds would display significantly more approach and fewer avoidance behaviors than a matched control group placed on standard isolette mattresses.

METHOD

Subjects

Twenty-two premature infants, 29-33 weeks gestational age at birth, were randomly assigned by pairs to either the control or experimental group. Sixteen were patients at one hospital's neonatal intensive care unit, and the remaining six were patients at the neonatal intensive care unit of a hospital in another city in the same state. Infants were selected and assigned to groups as they became available over a three-month period. A total of 15 male and 7 female subjects were recruited, with 7 males and 4 females in the experimental group and 8 males and 3 females in the control group. Informed consent was obtained from the parents of each infant prior to participation in the study.

Participation in the study occurred within the first two weeks of life, and, at the time of the study, the infants ranged from 30-34 weeks postconceptional age. All infants were appropriate in weight for gestational age, were receiving intermittent oral gavage feedings, and were free of major medical complications. Infants with mild respiratory distress syndrome (RDS), apnea of prematurity, mildly increased bilirubin, and mild hypoglycemia were included. Infants with moderate to severe RDS or severe postnatal complications, infants who were small or large for gestational age, and infants requiring surgery or ventilatory support for more than one week were excluded. All infants were breathing room air at the time of observation.

Apparatus

The waterbed used was the Medpro Neo-Float Neonatal Floatation System* with oscillating, dual frequency rhythmic wave stimulator. It consists of a water chamber which is filled with 3.75 liters of water and

---

*Medpro, Inc., 275 Highway 18, East Brunswick, New Jersey 08816.

rests on top of a plexiglass platform within an air-filled frame. The 14 × 25 × 2 inch foam mattress with a vinyl surface is covered with a disposable, waterproof, fitted mattress cover; is inserted in a pillow case; and is covered with a blanket. Oscillations are mechanically provided at 16 +/− 4 pulsations per minute by air pulses through an inflation bladder which is placed between the water chamber and platform. Temperature of the waterbed is maintained by the isolette heating system.

Procedure

Immediately after gavage feeding, infants in the experimental group were placed in the prone position on a waterbed. The period immediately following gavage feeding was chosen as the treatment/observation period for this study for two reasons. First, as an invasive procedure, gavage feeding is considered to have a disorganizing effect on motor behavior, therefore, during this period the proposed effects of waterbed use may be of most benefit to the infants. Second, preliminary observations during a pilot study indicated that the amount of motor activity in premature infants in general seemed greater in the period immediately after feeding.

To ensure equal handling between treatment and control groups, infants in the control group were picked up and then placed back onto their standard isolette mattresses in the prone position before and after each observation. The infants in the treatment group were returned to their original isolettes and mattresses following the one half hour observation period while on the waterbed mattress. This procedure was repeated for each infant after each of five consecutive feedings in one day.

Data were collected by direct behavioral observation using a time sampling technique. The dependent variables were chosen from two categories of behavior, approach and avoidance, from the Assessment of Premature Infant Behavior regulation catalogue.[33] Approach behaviors (also termed groping behaviors)[33] are defined as those that increase the organism's reception of contact with stimuli. These behaviors can be oriented toward self, as in hand-to-mouth, or they can be oriented toward other sources of stimulation in the environment. Avoidance behaviors are those that reduce contact with stimulation. For this study, one approach behavior (hand-to-mouth) and five avoidance behaviors (grimace, startle, trunkal arch, finger splay, salute) were examined. Each behavior was operationally defined as follows:

1. *Hand-to-mouth* Infant brings hand or fingers to the perioral area. Infant does not have to be successful at reaching the mouth but should reach the perioral area, which includes the cheeks, chin, nose, and lips. The infant must move into this position; remaining in the same position does not qualify.

2. *Grimace* The infant's face is distorted with lip and cheek retraction. Eye-brow knitting may occur but is not the sole component. A quality of tension or stress can be observed.
3. *Startle* A sudden total body "jerk" occurs; it is often, but not necessarily, associated with or followed by extensive trunk and limb movement. Sudden movement of an individual limb does not qualify.
4. *Trunkal arch* The infant's trunk arches or head extends in an arching fashion (past neutral position). Associated limb movement may occur, but extremities do not have to extend. The infant may show stiffening or straightening of the trunk, retraction of the shoulder blades, wrinkling of the skin on the back, or hyperextension of the neck.
5. *Finger splay* The infant's hand(s) open strongly. The fingers on one or both hands are extended and separated from each other.
6. *Salute* Arms or legs are suddenly fully extended either singly or simultaneously. Salute often involves full extension of the limb into mid-air, but in prone the distal portion of the limb might not go fully into mid-air.

A tape recording was used as a timing device during the observation periods. One hundred 10-second "observe" intervals alternated with 7.5-second "record" intervals during the observation periods (29.1 minutes). One or more occurrences of any of the preselected behaviors during each 10-second interval resulted in a score of 1 for that behavior. The dependent measure for statistical analysis consisted of the sum of the intervals marked 1 for each behavior across the five observation periods.

Interobserver reliability was established by the first author and a neonatal nurse, both of whom have had extensive experience in working with premature infants. Independent observations of the dependent variables were made on a randomly selected subset of observations. Throughout the period of the study, these independent observations were made on half of the subjects at both hospitals (six control and five experimental infants). Reliability was determined for each group by calculating the number of agreements divided by the sum of the number of agreements plus disagreements for both occurrence and non-occurrence of each behavior. The percentage of agreement for the six behaviors ranged from 80 to 100% in the experimental group and from 85 to 95% in the control group. The percentage of agreement for non-occurrence of the six behaviors ranged from 98 to 100% across the two groups.

Two-tailed t-tests were used to compare all pre-treatment data, and one-tailed t-tests were used to compare treatment and control groups on each of the six behaviors. The traditional alpha level of .05 was established for determining statistical significance.

RESULTS

In order to confirm the comparability of experimental and control groups based on group composition and subject criteria, an analysis of selected pre-treatment characteristics was performed. Results of a two-tailed t-test indicated no significant differences between control and experimental groups on the variables presented in Table 1. Analyses were completed on all six dependent variables using hospital as the independent variable. No indication of differences among subjects as a function of hospital was noted, therefore subjects from the two hospitals were grouped together.

The means and standard deviations of occurrence of each of the dependent variables as a function of group are presented in Table 2. Results of one-tailed t-tests to compare the mean scores of the experimental and control groups on each behavior indicated highly significant differences between groups on five out of six variables. As hypothesized, the frequency

TABLE 1

Infant Pretreatment Variables as a Function of Group

Variable	Treatment Group		Control Group	
	X̄	SD*	X̄	SD
Gestational Age at birth (wks)	31.31	0.90	31.27	1.47
Gestational Age at study (wks)	32.50	0.94	32.40	1.48
Birth Weight (gm)	1474.09	164.63	1568.00	200.86
Weight at study (gm)	1345.90	165.48	1473.90	219.90
Apgar at 1 minute	7.30	1.56	7.36	2.11
Apgar at 5 minutes	8.70	0.67	8.54	1.03
Duration of ventilatory assistance (days)	1.00	1.26	0.81	1.83
Duration of supplementary oxygen (days)	1.81	1.47	2.72	3.25
Duration of phototherapy	2.18	2.08	1.90	1.37

* SD = standard deviation

TABLE 2

Group Comparison of Dependent Variables

| | Treatment Group | | Control Group | | t values |
	X̄	SD	X̄	SD	(one-tailed)
hand-to-mouth	23.00	5.95	8.81	5.19	5.96*
grimace	23.09	17.13	54.00	19.78	-3.92*
startle	2.81	3.48	11.45	5.48	-4.41*
trunkal arch	14.36	7.63	36.00	14.24	-4.44*
finger splay	20.54	17.13	23.72	13.83	-0.48 n.s.
salute	23.36	12.86	71.36	27.39	-5.26*

n.s. = not significant
*   = $p < .001$

of occurrence of hand-to-mouth was significantly greater in the experimental than the control group. In addition, the frequencies of occurrence of four out of the five avoidance behaviors (grimace, startle, trunkal arch, and salute) were significantly greater in the control group than the experimental group. No significant difference between experimental and control groups was found in the frequency of one behavior, finger splay.

As can be seen from Table 2 very large differences between means were found on each of the five behaviors that showed statistical significance. In fact, the means of each of these behaviors are at least twice as large in favor of the experimental group.

DISCUSSION

The immediate effects of waterbed flotation are demonstrated by this study, and with one exception (finger splay), the original hypotheses are confirmed. The results of this study demonstrate that, following gavage feeding of relatively healthy premature infants, a particular type of waterbed stimulation makes hand-to-mouth behavior much more likely while simultaneously decreasing the likelihood of four avoidance behaviors. These results support clinical observations made during previous neonatal waterbed research which suggested that movements of premature infants on waterbeds are less random and more modulated with less frequent startles and more hand-to-mouth contact.[20]

Recent models of infant development propose that infants are active participants within their environments.[26-30] The current study further supports these views of infant abilities by illustrating the capacity of the premature infants placed on waterbeds to organize their own behaviors and make adaptive responses. One could argue that *decreases* in avoidance behavior, as seen in this study, may not be representative of adaptive behavior because the occurrence of avoidance responses (as in withdrawal from overstimulation or noxious stimuli) is adaptive. In this study, however, no known noxious stimuli were immediately present during the observation periods. Furthermore, although dependent variables may not be statistically compared to each other, the control group's performance seems to show that avoidance behaviors occurred frequently, while hand-to-mouth behavior was relatively infrequent. This indicates that the infants in this study were not prevented from making avoidance responses. Though the optimal balance between approach and avoidance behaviors in premature infants is not known, a universal practice of infant care is to soothe infants whose movements appear restless and erratic. The oscillating waterbed environment, initially developed for premature infants because of its similarity to the intrauterine environment,[20] appears to have this soothing effect without impairing the infants' responsiveness to the environment.

Therapists' abilities to affect the organizational systems of developing infants through monitoring or changing sensory experience may have far-reaching effects on various developmental processes. For example, waterbed stimulation might be of benefit in promoting parent-infant bonding. Kennell and Klaus[34] have stated that prematurity challenges or threatens the bonding process since the parents often have difficulty perceiving the responsiveness of their premature infant to stimulation. If waterbed stimulation increases approach behaviors and reduces avoidance behaviors, then it might be used in conjunction with other techniques to enhance social responsiveness of the premature infant and thus stimulate the social reciprocity which is foundational for bonding.

Other implications of this study relate to the care of premature infants under clinical conditions which are especially stress-inducing. The soothing effect of waterbed flotation might be useful to infants in traumatic situations, such as after surgery or other medical procedures. Some authors have pointed out that newborn intensive care units actually bombard infants with meaningless, uncoordinated sensory stimuli that might disrupt normal diurnal rhythms.[35-36] Investigations should be made to determine whether the effects of the waterbeds are to cushion and thereby subdue, or to enhance extraneous stimuli such as noise. Certainly waterbeds provide an opportunity for eliciting coordinated movements and may be a source of self- or other-produced rhythmic input. Finally, health care professionals who are involved in assessment of infant behavior might also consider the possibility that infants perform better in terms of behavioral organization if they have been on a waterbed.

Whatever the short-term or long-term developmental effects of waterbed flotation, this study adds evidence that this type of stimulation is relevant to premature infants, at least following gavage feeding. Several authors[1-4] have reviewed the effects of various types of sensory stimulation on premature infants and have suggested the need for greater understanding of how different types of sensory stimuli affect different types of responses in premature infants. The logical direction of further studies in this area would be toward more specifically identifying the stimulus dimensions responsible for the effects of waterbed flotation on infant behavior and development. Although previous waterbed research has implicated the vestibular-proprioceptive system in mediating the effects of waterbed flotation, no one sensory system has yet been isolated. Waterbed stimulation includes containment, warmth, touch, and kinesthetic, vestibular, and proprioceptive input. Many sensory modalities are known to have some influence on such processes as muscle tone, sensorimotor functions, and arousal,[37-39] and any of these influences could underlie some of the changes seen in this study. Furthermore, a waterbed provides contingent feedback to the infant's movements. Are the effects seen in this study the result of vestibular stimulation, some other dimension of the waterbed, or an interaction among dimensions?

Another direction for future studies is to elaborate and expand on the response variables investigated in this study. We noted through informal observation during this study that clinical variables besides those formally investigated, may have been affected by waterbed stimulation. For example, while the observers were recording frequency of hand-to-mouth behaviors, they noted that the duration of maintained hand-to-mouth behavior seemed greater in the infants on waterbeds. Posture may also have been affected by the waterbed, since the experimental infants seemed to maintain greater flexion over a greater portion of time than did the control infants. These observations have not been experimentally verified and suggest future investigations, which might also explore the effects of waterbed stimulation on muscle tone, specific motor functions, or more complex processes involving sensorimotor skills or learning.

REFERENCES

1. Field, TM: Supplemental stimulation of preterm neonates. *Early Hum Dev* 4:301-314, 1980
2. Masi W: Supplemental stimulation of the premature infant, in Field TM (ed): *Infants Born at Risk.* New York, SP Medical and Scientific Books, 1979
3. Schaefer M, Hatcher RP, Barglow PD: Prematurity and infant stimulation: A review of research. *Child Psychiatry Hum Dev* 10: 199-212, 1980
4. Touwen BCL: The preterm infant in the extrauterine environment: Implications for neurology. *Early Hum Dev* 4: 287-300, 1980

5. Langworthy OR: Development of behavior patterns and myelinization of the nervous system in the human fetus and infant. *Contrib Embryol* 24: 3-57, 1933

6. Erway L: Otolith formation and trace elements: A theory of schizophrenic behavior. *J Orthomol Psychiatry* 4: 16-26, 1975

7. Korner AF, Kraemer HC, Haffner ME et al.: Effects of waterbed flotation on premature infants: A pilot study. *Pediatrics* 56: 361-367, 1975

8. Neal MV: Organizational behavior of the premature infant. *Birth Defects* 15: 43-60, 1979

9. Clark DL, Kreutzberg JR, Chee FKW: Vestibular stimulation influence on motor development in infants. *Science* 196: 1228-1229, 1977

10. Gregg C, Haffner M, Korner AF: The relative efficacy of vestibular-proprioceptive stimulation and the upright position in enhancing visual pursuit in neonates. *Child Dev* 47: 309-314, 1976

11. Freedman D, Boverman H: The effects of kinesthetic stimulation on certain aspects of development in premature infants. *Am J Orthopsychiatry* 36: 223-224, 1966

12. Korner AF, Thoman EB: The relative efficacy of contact and vestibular-proprioceptive stimulation on the activity of two-month-old infants. *Child Dev* 43: 443-453, 1972

13. Pederson D, Ter Vrugt D: The influence of amplitude and frequency of vestibular stimulation on the activity of two-month-old infants. *Child Dev* 44: 122-128, 1973

14. Harlow H: The nature of love. *Am Psychol* 13: 673-685, 1958

15. Mason WA: Early social deprivation in the non-human primate: Implications for human behavior in environmental influences, in Glass DC (ed): *Environmental Influences.* New York, Rockefeller University Press & Russell Sage Foundation, 1968

16. Thoman EV, Korner AF: Effects of vestibular stimulation on the behavior and development of infant rats. *Dev Psychol* 5: 92-98, 1971

17. Neal MV: The relationship between a regimen of vestibular stimulation and the developmental behavior of the premature infant. *Nurs Res* 17: 568-569, 1968

18. Barnard KE: The effect of stimulation on the duration and amount of sleep and wakefulness in the premature infant. *Dissert Abstr Internat* 33: 2167B, 1972

19. Rose SA: Enhancing visual recognition memory in preterm infants. *Dev Psychol* 16: 85-96, 1980

20. Korner AF: Maternal rhythms and waterbeds: A form of intervention with premature infants, in Thoman EB (ed): *Origins of the Infant's Social Responsiveness.* Hillsdale, NJ, Lawrence Erlbaum Associates, 1979

21. Korner, AF, Guilleminault C, Van den Hoed J et al.: Reduction of sleep apnea and bradycardia in preterm infants on oscillating waterbeds: A controlled polygraphic study. *Pediatrics* 61: 528-533, 1978

22. Korner AF, Ruppel, EM, Rho JM: Effects of waterbeds on the sleep and motility of theophylline-treated preterm infants. *Pediatrics* 70: 864-869, 1982

23. Kramer LI, Pierpont, ME: Rocking waterbed and auditory stimulation to enhance growth of preterm infants. *Pediatrics* 88: 297-299, 1976

24. Burns KA: Developmental progress in premature infants as a function of oscillating waterbed and auditory stimulation. *Dissert Abstr Internat* 41: 4281B, 1981

25. Als H, Tronick F, Adamson L et al.: The behavior of the full-term infant. *Dev Med Child Neurol* 18: 590-602, 1976

26. Als H, Lester BM, Brazelton TB: Dynamics of the behavioral organization of the premature infant: A theoretical perspective, in Field TM (ed): *Infants Born at Risk,* New York, SP Medical and Scientific Books, 1979

27. Brazelton TB, Parker WB, Zuckerman B: The importance of neonatal behavior. *Curr Probl Pediatr* 7: 1-82, 1976

28. Lipsitt LP: The pleasures and annoyances of infants: Approach and avoidance behavior, in Thoman EB (ed): *Origins of the Infant's Social Responsiveness.* Hillsdale, NJ, Lawrence Erlbaum Associates, 1979

29. Brazelton TB: *Neonatal Behavioral Assessment Scale,* Clinics in Developmental Medicine, No. 50, Philadelphia, JB Lippincott, 1973

30. Dubowitz LMS, Dubowitz V: *The Neurological Assessment of the Preterm and Full-term Newborn Infant,* Clinics in Developmental Medicine, No. 79, Philadelphia, JB Lippincott, 1981

31. Korner SF: Conceptual issues in infancy research, in Osofsky JD (ed): *Handbook of Infant Development.* New York, John Wiley & Sons, 1979

32. Als H, Lester BM, Tronick E et al.: Manual for the assessment of preterm infant behavior

(APIB), in Fitzgerald HE, Lester EM, Yogman MW (eds): *Theory and Research in Behavioral Pediatrics,* vol 2. New York, Plenum Publishing Corp, 1982, pp 65-133

33. Als H, Lester BM, Tronick EC et al.: Towards a research instrument for the assessment of preterm infants' behavior (APIB), in Fitzgerald HE, Lester BM, Yogman MW (eds): *Theory and Research in Behavioral Pediatrics,* vol 2. New York, Plenum Publishing Corp, 1982

34. Kennell JH, Klaus MH: Caring for the parents of premature or sick infants, in MH Klaus & JH Kennell (eds): *Parent-Infant Bonding.* St. Louis, MO, CV Mosby, 1982

35. Newman LF: Social and sensory environment of low birth weight infants in a special care nursery: An anthropological investigation. *J Nerv Ment Dis* 169: 448-455, 1981

36. Gottfried AW, Wallace-Lande P, Sherman-Brown S et al.: Physical and social environment of newborn infants in special care units. *Science* 214: 673-675, 1981

37. Martin JP: Role of the vestibular system in the control of posture and movement in man, in de Reuck AVS, Knight J (eds): *Myotatic, Kinesthetic and Vestibular Mechanisms,* Boston, Little, Brown & Co, 1966

38. Ayres AJ: *Sensory Integration and Learning Disorders.* Los Angeles, Western Psychological Services, 1972

39. Noback CR: *The Human Nervous System: Basic Principles of Neurobiology.* New York, McGraw-Hill Book Co, 1981

Effects of Controlled Rotary Vestibular Stimulation on the Motor Performance of Infants with Down Syndrome

Joan Snyder Lydic, ScD, LPT
Mary Margaret Windsor, MEd, OTR
Margaret A. Short, PhD, OTR
Terry Ann Ellis, MS, OTR

ABSTRACT. Eighteen infants, ranging in age from four to ten months at the onset of the study, were divided into control and treatment groups using a stratified random sampling procedure. Children were selected on the basis of age, specific type of Down syndrome, and participation in a regular sensorimotor intervention program from outside the study. Children in the treatment group received, in their home, rotary vestibular stimulation three times weekly for twelve weeks in addition to their regular program. Children in the control group received only their regular program. All children were evaluated initially, at the end of six weeks, and at the end of twelve weeks by the same examiner, who was naive to group assignment. Evaluations included the Movement Assessment of Infants (MAI) and the Gross Motor section of the revised Peabody Developmental Motor Scales (PDMS).

Analyses of variance indicated significant trials but non-significant groups or interaction effects with both motor instruments. The hypothesized differential treatment effect of vestibular stimulation was not substantiated, but important clinical information was obtained. This study demonstrated that, over a 12-week period, Down syndrome infants are capable of making significant changes in motor abilities, to which both the Movement Assessment of Infants and the Peabody Developmental Motor Scales are sensitive. Treatment and control groups made equivalent changes. Whether those changes are the result of maturational variables

Joan Snyder Lydic is Adjunct Associate Professor of Physical Therapy, Departments of Allied Health Sciences and Health Administration, Southwest Texas State University, San Marcos, TX 78666. This study was conducted as part of the requirements for completion of the Doctor of Science degree at Boston University, Sargent College of Allied Health Professions, Boston, MA. Mary Margaret Windsor is in private practice in the Dover, NH area. Margaret A. Short was in private practice in Boston, MA at the time this study was done and is currently practicing in Saratoga Springs, NY. Terry Ann Ellis is in private practice in Boston, MA.

The authors wish to acknowledge Dr. David L. Nelson's assistance with research design and methodology and Dr. Kevin Nugent's suggestions regarding the parents' checklist designed for this study.

characteristic of Down syndrome infants at that age, family variables, or participation in early intervention programs is not known but is worth continued examination.

INTRODUCTION

Over 2,300 different genetic disorders exist, one of which is represented by a group of symptoms collectively referred to as Down syndrome.[1] Occurring once in every 600 to 700 live births, Down syndrome includes the most common type of mental retardation, and affects the total development of the individual.[2] As a result of the prevalence of Down syndrome and the profoundly disruptive effects it has on motor development, physical and occupational therapists often are asked to assume prominent roles in designing and implementing therapeutic programs for children exhibiting this syndrome. The types of techniques used in these interventions vary tremendously, and the efficacy of specific techniques is often either undocumented or ambiguous. Consequently, a therapist must rely heavily on previous clinical experience to determine the choice of intervention techniques. Systematic evaluation of the parameters of different interventions which are successful with children of specific disabilities would help ensure more consistent and reliable foundations for therapy.[3]

Of particular interest to the therapist treating the child with Down syndrome is remediation of those characteristics which are thought to hinder motor abilities: hypotonicity and hypermobility,[4-13] delayed or persistent primitive reflexes,[13-16] slow or irregular attainment of normal, mature postural reactions,[13] and paucity of refined movement as evidenced by abnormal patterns lacking the more qualitative aspects of movement such as rotation along the body axis.[17,18]

Many investigators have reported positive effects of intervention on gross and fine motor development of children with Down syndrome,[19-25] and others have indicated specific exercises which are thought to foster the abilities of this population.[26-36] In contrast to these reported positive effects, Harris[37] found no statistically significant enhancement of the motor abilities of infants with Down syndrome who received neurodevelopmental therapy in addition to their regular infant stimulation program when they were compared to similar children who received only the infant stimulation. Harris attributed these non-significant results to the small sample size (N = 20) and the inability of the measurement instruments, the Bayley Scales of Infant Development[38] and the Peabody Developmental Motor Scales (1974 edition),[39] to detect subtle changes in the motor abilities of young infants with Down syndrome.

Many different assessment tools have been used in studies examining the motor abilities of Down syndrome children ranging in age from 2.7 to 129 months of age. These tests include: the Bayley Scales of Infant Development,[40-45] the Gesell Developmental Schedules,[20,43,46,47] the Peabody Developmental Motor Scales,[45,48,49] and the Movement Assessment of Infants.[49] Although these tools have proven sensitive enough to reflect changes in motor abilities, they have not been consistently tested for the degree to which they can detect qualitative or subtle motor changes which might appear during, or as a result of, intervention. In an attempt to provide such information about two tests, Lydic, Short and Nelson compared the Movement Assessment of Infants (MAI)[50] with the earlier version of the Peabody Developmental Motor Scales (PDMS).[39] Both tests were administered to ten Down syndrome infants at the beginning and end of a six week period. Comparisons of the test results suggested that, when compared to the PDMS, the MAI was more sensitive to developmental changes and appeared more stable over time. PDMS scores did reflect greater variance than did MAI scores, but the authors were unable to determine if the variance was a reflection of test sensitivity to individual differences or of error. Lydic and colleagues pointed out that the new revision of the PDMS[51] includes standardized instructions which would reduce error variance in test administration. Comparisons between the MAI and the newly revised PDMS have not been conducted.

In spite of the potential insensitivity of many assessments to subtle motor changes over time, study results have consistently demonstrated remediative effects of vestibular stimulation on the motor abilities of children, including those who have Down syndrome. In general, vestibular stimulation in various forms has been found effective in enhancing visual alertness and tracking,[52-54] increasing weight gain and mental functioning,[55-57] causing soothing or increasing arousal.[58-62] Specifically, with regard to gross motor abilities, vestibular stimulation has been shown to be effective in fostering reflex integration and motor development in normal infants,[63,64] premature infants,[53,55,65] in children with cerebral palsy,[66,67] and in children who are mentally retarded.[48,68]

What specific populations benefit the most and which parameters of vestibular input are most successful are not clear. The findings of studies by Kantner and colleagues[68] and Ottenbacher and colleagues,[48] however, point to the possibility that controlled rotary vestibular stimulation may be especially effective in promoting the motor development of infants displaying some of the characteristics associated with Down syndrome. For example, over a two-week period, Kantner and colleagues provided rotary vestibular stimulation to Down syndrome and normal intelligence infants ranging in age from 6 to 24 months. The child with Down syndrome and the normal children in the treatment group all displayed improvements in motor performance and evidence of greater vestibular habituation than the control group. Similarly, positive changes after vestibular stimulation were reported by Ottenbacher, Short and Watson.[48] In this study, Ottenbacher and colleagues investigated the effects of a clinically applied program of vestibular input on the neuromotor performance of a group of 38 developmentally disabled children ranging in age from 39 to 129 months. Analyses revealed that, when compared to controls who received only the sensorimotor program, subjects who were treated with 13 weeks of vestibular stimulation, in addition to their regular sensorimotor therapy program, made significantly greater gains in gross motor and fine motor development, as measured by the earlier version of the PDMS, and in measures of reflex integration. Of particular relevance to the present study were the findings that greater gains were seen in the younger, low muscle-tone children than in the older children who displayed spasticity.

The general consensus from the majority of studies is that vestibular stimulation is effective in remediating developmental delays, however, some studies do not support these findings.[69,70] Casler[69] found no significant differences between groups of institutionalized infants who received vestibular and auditory stimulation and those who did not. Likewise, Sellick and Over[70] question the efficacy of vestibular stimulation. In an examination of cerebral-palsied children placed in either a vestibular stimulation treatment group or an untreated control group, Sellick and Over reported no differences between groups on the Bayley Scales of Infant Development. The authors suggested that discrepancies in documented benefits of vestibular stimulation might be avoided if future investigators of any type of intervention take greater care with methodological issues. These methodological requirements for evaluating therapeutic techniques are relevant to the present study. They include: (1) experimental design using treatment and control groups, (2) clearly defined population from which the sample is drawn, (3) objective assessment measures, (4) assessment of performance across time, and (5) employment of blind methodology.

The present study is a further investigation into the effects of vestibular stimulation on the motor abilities of developmentally delayed infants. We attempted to clarify some of the conflicting findings regarding vestibular stimulation and intervention with Down syndrome infants. Many of the suggestions and relevant findings of the previously discussed experiments have been incorporated here. For example, subjects for this study were selected from a homogeneous developmentally disabled population (Down syndrome), which is commonly treated by physical and occupational therapists and which displays characteristics similar to those remediated in other studies.[e.g., 48,64,68] The specific form of intervention used in this study is one which is often used in the clinical treatment of developmentally delayed children, which has previously been reported to enhance the motor abilities of those children, and which has potential use in non-laboratory settings, such as the home or clinic.

This study was designed to examine systematically, over repeated measures, the motor effects of vestibular stimulation when it was used as part of a therapeutic program. The majority of the criteria suggested by Sellick and Over[70] were addressed in this study and, for clarity and replication, thorough definitions are provided for the parameters (frequency, duration and speed) of therapy as well as the equipment, handling and positioning used as a part of intervention. Finally, dependent variables were selected based on their previous demonstration of sensitivity to changes occurring as a result of vestibular stimulation[48] or for their ability to reflect developmental changes in the specific types of subjects selected for this study.[49]

METHOD

Subjects

Twenty infants, ten males and ten females, with Down syndrome served as subjects for this study. Before the third and final evaluation, two males dropped out of the study because of family problems which made their continued participation too difficult for the parent. The 18 children for which data are reported, ranged in age from approximately four to ten months of age at the time of initial testing. Ottenbacher and colleagues[48] demonstrated that the largest motor gains in response to vestibular stimulation occurred in younger, low-toned subjects. Similarly, Kantner and colleagues[68] demonstrated positive effects of vestibular stimulation in young normal intelligence and in Down syndrome infants. Thus, in the present study, young infants with Down syndrome were selected in order to maximize the chance of obtaining significant effects of vestibular stimulation.

Some constraints on the ages of the infants were necessary because of the measuring instruments selected for this study. The MAI is not reliable for children under four months of age,[71] and can only be used with children up to twelve months of age when the children are scoring age-appropriately. Children selected for this study, therefore, could be no younger than three months nor older than ten months at the beginning of testing.

To control for the possible differences in children with the three types of Down syndrome, only those children with Trisomy 21, confirmed by chromosomal testing, were selected as subjects. Children who had major medical problems, such as uncorrected cardiac problems, were excluded. In addition to the present study, all children were participating in an intervention program which included sensorimotor training, which took place either in the home or in a clinic or other facility.

Subjects were initially recruited by contacting all early intervention programs in the State of Massachusetts. A letter describing the study and the need for subjects was mailed to each program, and a follow-up telephone call was made to each director. In addition, a presentation made by the senior author to a state conference for early intervention programs described the previous work of several of the authors, the clinical findings regarding the motor behaviors of children with Down syndrome, the proposal and the need for subjects for the current study. When only two referrals were obtained after five months, a second letter was mailed to the same early intervention programs. In addition, contact was made for recruiting subjects from other state agencies as well as national and regional organizations serving individuals with Down syndrome. Agencies and one parent desirous of additional information were sent packets of literature including: an annotated bibliography of motor development in Down syndrome children,[72] three review articles[3,73,74] regarding vestibular stimulation, one article[48] describing the positive effects of vestibular stimulation, and a copy of the proposal for this study.

Over the fourteen month period in which subjects were recruited, 20 Down syndrome children, who met the criteria for selection, and whose parents were willing to participate, were located from the states of Massachusetts, New Hampshire, Ohio, and West Virginia. Parental permission for participation of the infants in this study was obtained for all subjects, and, at all times, the researchers in this study made efforts to be sensitive to parental concerns.

Instruments

The Movement Assessment of Infants[50] and the Gross Motor section of the revised Peabody Developmental Motor Scales[51] were used to measure the motor abilities of the infants with Down syndrome who participated in this investigation. Both of these tools were selected in order to extract information about changes in muscle tone, reflexes, and other developmental data; to use norm-referenced tests, and because of their previous demonstrated sensitivity in detecting the more qualitative, often subtle, motor changes in infants with Down syndrome.[49] The clinical experience of the senior author plus the results of many studies[e.g., 2,13-15,17,18,75,76] suggest that the two motor areas likely to be deficient in Down syndrome children are tone and postural reactions. The MAI permits assessment of these areas in addition to volitional movement and primitive reflexes. The overall score on this assessment tool reflects a developmental at-risk factor.

Although the MAI appears to be ideal for evaluating the motor abilities of infants with Down syndrome, it is normed only for four-month-old children. Thus, to provide norm-references and to strengthen the assessment component of this study, the PDMS was also used. In the latest version,[51] the authors of the PDMS suggest that the instrument can be reliably used with normal individuals as well as those with developmental disabilities. Although this assessment does have weaknesses,[77] its original version[39] was effective in detecting motoric changes in developmentally delayed, especially low-toned, children exposed to vestibular stimulation.[48] Thus, use of the PDMS seemed appropriate for the Down syndrome infants in this study.

Scoring on the MAI and the PDMS is different. Unlike MAI scores which decrease with age, scores on the PDMS increase with age. In the present study, raw scores on the PDMS were not converted to motor quotients so that easy comparisons could be made with the raw scores from the MAI.

Apparatus

A commercially available A-frame, with a swivel hook center at the top allowed attachment of a commercially available wooden seat (Figure 1) or net hammock (Figure 2) in which the subjects were positioned for

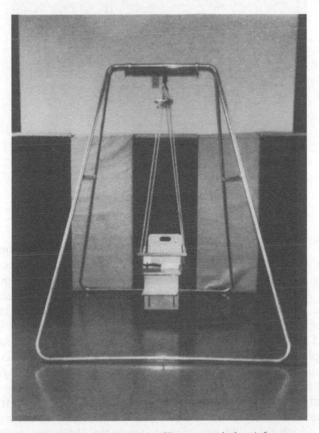

FIGURE 1. Wooden swing-like seat attached to A-frame.

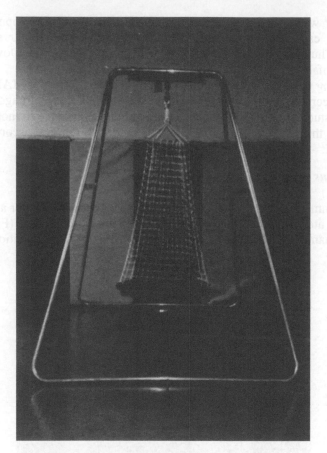

FIGURE 2. Net hammock with vinyl pad.

treatment. The wooden seat with a safety dowel across the front had an adjustable one-piece leg rest and an adjustable one-piece footrest, as well as a safety strap that was fastened at a level straight back from the hips of the child. Additionally, foam padding was used to ensure the seated position of the child with 90 degrees of hip flexion, 90 degrees of knee flexion, and 90 degrees of ankle flexion (Figure 3). For the smaller infants, a cardboard insert was placed inside the seat and secured. A small infant could be placed in the insert within the seat and remain in correct position for treatment; without the insert, the position changed. The nylon net hammock had dowel rods at the top through which the ends were tied onto a metal ring; the ring was attached to the swivel hook on the A-frame. Inside the net was a vinyl-covered foam pad (62 cm long, 44 cm wide, 2 cm thick) on which the child was placed. Once the child was positioned in supine flexion, the cuddling effect of the net hammock, caused by its end being pulled together, helped to maintain this position (Figure 4).

Procedures

After parental consent was obtained for the subjects, a letter including appreciation for participation and an explanation of the importance of the study was mailed to the children's parents. Each child was then evaluated by the same examiner. This examiner as well as three therapists (interveners) performing the vestibular intervention were clinically certified and familiar with current research regarding the motor development of Down syndrome children and the clinical effects of vestibular stimulation. The examiner, who was experienced in the uses and administration

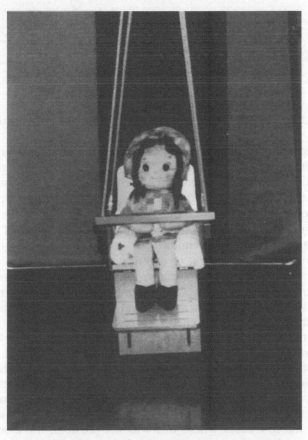

FIGURE 3. Positioning used for infants in the seat.

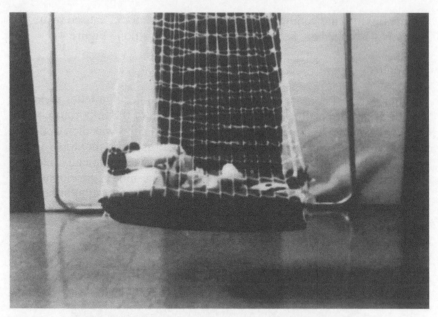

FIGURE 4. Positioning used for infants in the net hammock.

of the MAI and the PDMS, was naive to all group assignments throughout the study.

A counterbalanced procedure for administration of the instruments was used to control for order effects. Order of administration of the instruments was randomly determined for the first child and every subsequent odd-numbered child. The order of test administration for the second child and each even-numbered child was reversed from that of the previous one. This randomization procedure was followed for each of the three assessment periods for each child.

Assignment to the treatment or control groups was performed using a stratified random sampling procedure. The first child of a particular age between four and ten months was randomly assigned to one group. The next child of the same age was automatically assigned to the other group, thus forming two groups matched for age.

At the time of testing, all children were in the quiet alert state described by Brazelton.[78] To maintain this state, considered to be optimal for eliciting the best performance of the child, comfort and soothing in the form of cuddling were provided by the examiner, or when necessary, by the parent. If needed, a rest period was allowed during the assessment period. Whenever possible, the assessments were administered in the children's homes. In the few cases where this was not possible, the examiner attempted to perform the testing in a site familiar to the children. Parents and other adult relatives were permitted to remain quietly in the room with the children during assessments.

After the initial assessment, the children in the treatment group received twelve weeks of vestibular stimulation. This stimulation, similar to that used by Ottenbacher and colleagues,[48] consisted of controlled rotary input in two positions in order to activate the otoliths and the semicircular canals. Each treatment child was first lifted by the intervener, who maintained the child's flexion and placed him or her upright in the wooden seat. The position of 90 degrees of hip, knee, and ankle flexion was maintained. The intervener, using headphones, listened to a tape recording of the procedure. This ensured a standard, consistent procedure used with each child.

Treatment began with one minute of spinning the child, clockwise, in the wooden seat for seventeen revolutions, manually provided as one continuous turn. A one-minute rest period followed. Then, the same procedure was repeated in a counter-clockwise direction. The child was then removed from the seat and placed on a mat or other comfortable surface. The net hammock was then suspended from the swivel hook, and the intervener placed the child in supine position with the knees flexed up and the arms across the chest. The same procedure of clockwise rotation, rest period, counter-clockwise rotation, was carried out. The entire intervention, including time required to set up equipment, lasted approximately 20 minutes.

The children's reactions to stimulation were closely monitored. The intervener was instructed to look for rapid changes in respiration rate, heart rate, and skin color as symptoms of intolerance to the intervention. If these symptoms occurred, the intervener would have discontinued stimulation that day, and subsequent intolerance would have resulted in discontinuing the subject from the study. No child was discontinued from the study for these reasons.

Controlled vestibular stimulation was given three times weekly for twelve weeks to children in the treatment group. Any child who missed more than four of the scheduled treatment sessions was dropped from the study. When schedule conflicts arose, new treatment times were rescheduled within the same week. All intervention was done in the home or in a familiar site. Because the A-frame was too heavy and cumbersome to be portable, a separate frame was placed at each intervention site. All other equipment was removed at the end of each session. In order to ensure that the examiner remained unaware of subjects' group assignment, the parents were instructed to refrain from discussing the intervention with the examiner. Similar instructions were given to the parents of the children in the control group.

A total of three evaluation sessions were conducted for all treatment and control children by an examiner unaware of group assignment, who administered the MAI and the PDMS before, after six weeks of treatment, and at the end of the twelve week program of intervention. At the time of each assessment, the parents completed an intervention checklist. Information from this form was used to detect other variables, like illness, that might affect the child's motor performance. In addition, the checklist included the parents' subjective impressions of changes in the child's motor abilities. During the entire study, children in both the treatment and control groups continued to receive, from other sources, regular sensorimotor therapy without rotary vestibular stimulation.

DATA ANALYSIS AND RESULTS

The level of significance for all analyses was pre-set at the conventional p = .05 in order to achieve an adequate balance between Type I and Type II errors.[79] Descriptive statistics were used to examine similarities and differences noted during visual inspection of the data. Mean ages of the groups were comparable (M = 6.78, SD = 2.28; M = 6.83, SD = 2.18).

Both assessment tools demonstrated the ability to reflect overall changes in motor abilities over time as indicated by a general decrease in MAI scores and an increase in PDMS scores (Table 1).

When Pearson product moment correlation coefficients were used to test the stability of each instrument across time, r values were highly significant not only across the repeated administrations of each tool but also between the two tools (Table 2). Other correlations revealed no significant sex effects, but since age correlated positively with the test scores, partial correlations were performed to adjust for age and rule out potential artifactual effects. Results of these analyses revealed similarly high correlations between the two tests and across repeated administrations of each test (Table 3).

Separate 2 × 3 (groups × trials) analyses of variance with one repeated measure were performed using the raw data from each assessment tool. Significant trials, but no significant groups nor groups × trial interactions were obtained on either analysis (Tables 4 & 5). Both treatment and control infants increased comparable amounts on both scales. Over the 12-week intervention period, subjects who received vestibular stimulation in addition to their regular sensorimotor programs increased 23.2 points and 26.6 points on the MAI and the PDMS, respectively. Subjects in the control group, receiving outside sensorimotor programs without rotary vestibular stimulation, made similar gains. They increased an average total of 26.0 points on the MAI and 22.1 points on the PDMS.

Tabulations of the parental responses on the checklist indicated possible sources of group dissimilarities based on the number of subject ill-

Table 1

Means and Standard Deviations on the Two

Assessment Tools Across Three Intervals

Assessment Tool

Group

	Movement Assessment of Infants					
	Initial		6-week		12-week	
	$\overline{X}$	SD	$\overline{X}$	SD	$\overline{X}$	SD
Control	147.11	14.86	134.11	17.45	121.11	12.38
Treatment	139.89	18.84	129.44	21.14	116.67	19.04

	Peabody Developmental Motor Scales*					
	Initial		6-week		12-week	
	$\overline{X}$	SD	$\overline{X}$	SD	$\overline{X}$	SD
Control	58.89	17.65	71.11	14.20	81.00	11.79
Treatment	61.22	23.67	73.33	19.79	87.78	17.61

* Gross Motor section.

nesses, the number of times the child received his or her other regular clinical intervention, and the professional training of the person administering this additional treatment. Five children in the control group and seven treatment children received additional clinical intervention once per week, however, four control children as opposed to one treatment child received twice weekly additional clinical intervention. Further, more control children received this additional intervention from trained personnel. For example, four infants in the treatment group and 3 infants in the control group received clinical intervention from a teacher. The remainder of the treatment infants received this intervention from a therapist (n = 2) or a trainer (n = 3) compared with five control children who received clinical treatment from a therapist and one from a trainer. Examination of the therapists' training indicated that all five of the therapists providing outside intervention for the control infants were trained in the Neurodevelopmental Treatment (NDT) approach advocated by the Bobaths.[80,81] Four of these five therapists were also certified in sensory

Table 2

Pearson Correlations of Repeated Scores on the

Movement Assessment of Infants (MAI) and the

Peabody Developmental Motor Scales (PDMS)

	Initial		6-Week		12-Week	
	MAI1	PDMS1	MAI2	PDMS2	MAI3	PDMS3
MAI1	1.00					
PDMS1	-0.89*	1.00				
MAI2	0.92*	-0.90*	1.00			
PDMS2	-0.89*	0.95*	-0.93*	1.00		
MAI3	0.78*	-0.72*	0.88*	-0.82*	1.00	
PDMS3	-0.78*	0.76*	-0.84 *	0.87*	-0.88*	1.00

*$p < .001$

integration, promoted by Ayres.[82,83] The two therapists providing outside intervention for the treatment infants were likewise certified in both NDT and sensory integration.

All children who completed the study were able to be tested at approximately six and twelve weeks from the initial evaluation, however parents of the treatment children reported more frequent and severe illnesses of their children at all three assessment periods than did the parents of controls. For example, illnesses reported for the treatment children included colds and viruses (n = 9), ear infections (n = 3), and a respiratory infection requiring hospitalization (n = 1). For the control children, the parents reported only colds (n = 4) except for one ear infection. Compared with reports of healthy children during 16 separate evaluations of controls, only two treatment children were reported on separate sessions as having been healthy during the previous six-week period.

Subjective parental and interveners' observations were noted and tallied. Five parents of treatment infants reported noticing increased alertness as their child's sign of improvement over six weeks of vestibular stimulation. No parent of a control child noted this sign. The interveners reported that, as evidenced by relaxed facial musculature and smiles (similar to those reported by Freedman and Boverman[55] and Korner and Thoman[58]), all but one child consistently enjoyed the rotary stimulation. The one exception was a child who required hospitalization for respiratory problems during the study; however, he was able to complete the number of intervention sessions required for inclusion in the study.

DISCUSSION

Comparison of the repeated mean motor scores of the treatment and control subjects in this study failed to demonstrate significant effects as a result of vestibular stimulation. Hypothesized was a groups × trials interaction such that the treatment and control groups would display similar

Table 3

Partial Correlations of Repeated Scores on the

Movement Assessment of Infants (MAI) and the

Peabody Developmental Motor Scales (PDMS)

	Initial		6-Week		12-Week	
	MAI1	PDMS1	MAI2	PDMS2	MAI3	PDMS3
MAI1	1.00					
PDMS1	-0.81*	1.00				
MAI2	0.92*	-0.83*	1.00			
PDMS2	-0.81*	0.90*	-0.89*	1.00		
MAI3	0.60	-0.49	0.79*	-0.68*	1.00	
PDMS3	-0.60	0.56	-0.72*	0.80*	-0.79*	1.00

*$p < .05$

Table 4

Analysis of Variance For Groups By Trials

On The Movement Assessment of Infants

Source of Variance	Sums of Squares	df	Mean Squares	F	p
Total	20618.83	53			
Between subjects	13720.17	17			
Conditions	400.17	1	400.17	.48	.50
Error b	13320.00	16	832.50		
Within subjects	6898.66	36			
Trials	5455.44	2	2727.72	61.39	.0001
Groups X Trials	21.44	2	10.72	.24	.79
Error w	1421.78	32	44.43		

motor abilities upon initial testing but diverge in their performances on the two subsequent tests. We hypothesized that, when compared to the control subjects, the motor performance of the treatment subjects would be enhanced, after either (or both) the 6 or 12-week period of vestibular stimulation. The results indicated that both groups displayed equivalent enhanced performance on both the MAI and the Gross Motor Scale of the PDMS.

Although this study did not accomplish one of its major purposes, which was to clarify some of the issues regarding the use of controlled vestibular stimulation with developmentally delayed infants, it had many other positive findings. These are relevant clinical and procedural points which are important to share with other therapists and researchers interested in measuring motor development in delayed populations and in exploring the parameters of effective vestibular intervention. Two important findings of this study result from the significant trials effect obtained with both the MAI and the Gross Motor section of the recently revised PDMS. The trials effects indicate that, at this age, Down syndrome infants are capable of significantly enhancing their motor scores over a twelve week period. Additionally, both the MAI and the PDMS were sensitive enough to reflect that change.

Regarding the insignificant groups × trials interaction in this study, two immediate interpretations are suggested. One interpretation is that the vestibular stimulation had no effect, and the other is that an effect was achieved, but that the dependent variables were not sensitive enough to measure it. Both of these interpretations bear discussion as do other, less obvious, but equally important interpretations. The possibility that vestibular stimulation in the form of controlled rotary input does not enhance the motor performance of Down syndrome infants is consistent with the results of Sellick and Over's[70] study of cerebral-palsied children. Both similarities and differences exist between this and Sellick and Over's study. Both experiments used rigor in their methodology and design, but they differ in the nature of their subjects' disabilities as well as the ages of the subjects and the parameters of stimulation. The present study examined the effects of 36 sessions of vestibular stimulation delivered over a 12-week period to Down syndrome infants who were positioned upright and supine. Sellick and Over examined an older population of children, positioned upright and sidelying, while receiving 16 sessions of vestibular stimulation during a 4-week period.

Ottenbacher[84] has already cautioned about the overinterpretation of Sellick and Over's negative findings. He discussed the possibility of

Table 5

Analysis of Variance For Groups By Trials
On The Peabody Developmental Motor Scales

Source of Variance	Sums of Squares	df	Mean Squares	F	p
Total	2089.33	53			
Between subjects	13944.00	17			
Conditions	192.67	1	192.67	.22	.64
Error b	13751.33	16	859.46		
Within subjects	6949.34	36			
Trials	5329.00	2	2664.50	54.67	.0001
Groups X Trials	60.78	2	30.39	.62	.54
Error w	1559.56	32	48.74		

Sellick and Over's committing a Type II error, that is rejecting the null hypothesis when it is false. Additional clinical concerns have been noted regarding Sellick and Over's investigation. For example, Harris[37] has previously suggested that the Bayley Scales of Infant Development (the dependent variable in Sellick and Over's study), is not sensitive enough to reflect changes in motor development as a result of short term experimental intervention. Another potential confound in Sellick and Over's study is their method of matching subjects who are dissimilar in muscle tone, e.g., spastic or athetoid subjects matched with hypotonic children. If, as Ottenbacher and colleagues have demonstrated, vestibular stimulation is more effective with hypotonic children, then Sellick and Over's matching procedure may have washed out significant treatment effects.

The possibility of a Type II error in the present study is high because of the small sample size and the previous lack of extensive reliability and validity tests of the measuring instruments, however, the differences between the treatment and control groups in this study are so small that power analysis may not fully explain these data. The conclusion is that, although both this study and that of Sellick and Over fail to support the treatment effects of vestibular stimulation, confounds exist in both studies. Thus, further examination of the variables and other literature is warranted.

For example, this study used an intervention modelled after the successful intervention used by Ottenbacher and associates.[48] The primary difference between these studies is the nature of the subject population. None of the children in the study by Ottenbacher and colleagues were diagnosed as Down syndrome. Thus, one possible reason why the present study reported no significant changes between treatment and control groups may be the nature of the subject pool, the age of the subjects, or an interaction of these two variables. All of the subjects in the present study were younger than any subjects previously used for testing the effects of rotary vestibular stimulation. In addition, all of the subjects exhibited low muscle tone as a result of Down syndrome. One suggestion is that the low tone and motor delays of infants with Down syndrome cannot be sufficiently altered by vestibular or other forms of intervention. This suggestion, however, is countered by the significant trials effects obtained for both treatment and control children participating in this study. This trials effect indicates that all of the infants in this study displayed motor changes over time.

The fact that trials effects were obtained with both dependent variables indicates that both test instruments were sensitive to motor changes in this population of Down syndrome infants. Previous investigations have questioned the abilities of some instruments to pick up subtle motor changes in developmentally delayed subjects.[20,37] The present study is important because it demonstrates the usefulness of two relatively new motor instruments as well as the ability of delayed children to demonstrate significant progress over time. Campbell[85] has reported that continued reliability studies are necessary for the relatively untested MAI, and Palisano and Lydic[77] and Lydic and colleagues[49] have indicated the necessity of examining the recently revised PDMS. This study provides pertinent data regarding both.

Highly significant correlations among repeated administrations of the MAI and the Gross Motor section of the PDMS as well as between the two tools suggest that both instruments are valid, consistent measures of Down syndrome infant abilities over time. This finding lends further support to the use of the newer MAI and the PDMS, which have been designed especially to examine motor abilities. The older, more commonly used tools such as the Bayley Scales of Motor Development[35] and the Gesell Development Schedules,[86] have been and certainly still are beneficial in assessing overall milestones; however, when one is especially interested in measuring specific motor abilities, the newer assessment tools are recommended by the results of this investigation.

Children in the control and in the treatment groups showed similar changes on mean motor scores on the PDMS at the 6-week and the 12-week assessment; however on the MAI, children demonstrated changes in raw motor scores twice as great at the 12-week assessment than at the 6-week assessment. This suggests that the MAI may have detected more qualitative refinement of motor abilities that comes with age as opposed to attainment of motor milestones. The mean age for children in both groups was slightly less than seven months. Since infants with Down syndrome usually are delayed in more mature postural reflexes that require refinement of components of movement,[13-15,45,71,75,76] assessments would be more likely to detect small increments of change after 12 weeks rather than six weeks. Longer range studies might pick up differential effects of vestibular stimulation on the treatment compared with the control group, thus future longitudinal studies should look for such interactions.

One possible explanation for the significant trials but insignificant interaction effects are that both the control and treatment children benefitted from stimulation extraneous to this experiment. Both groups were receiving sensorimotor intervention from outside sources, and their participation in early intervention programs may have been responsible for the exhibited motor gains. Thus, in regard to the vestibular stimulation provided here, one interpretation is that the input was insufficient or ineffective in enhancing motor changes beyond those which the infants were already exhibiting. An ideal experimental paradigm would have included an untreated control group, but ethics and clinical judgement prevented that possibility. In the future investigators may want to use more sophisticated designs which enable them to account for extraneous treatment effects in control groups.

Despite the lack of experimental findings regarding vestibular stimulation, the fact that the groups both displayed significant motor changes is clinically compelling. Determining whether the motor changes occurred as a result of maturational factors, environmental stimulation provided by the families, or participation in other early intervention programming was beyond the scope of this study. The parent checklist used in this study was developed to ensure that changes in motor performance were not occurring as a result of factors other than vestibular stimulation. The use of this checklist subsequently became a possible means of explaining the lack of differential effects between the treatment and control groups. Examination of the checklist indicated that some control children received more regular outside intervention than did the children in the treatment group. Additionally, twice as many children in the control group received regular intervention by a therapist with special training in Neurodevelopmental Therapy or sensory integration.

In the dynamic treatment advocated in the NDT approach described by Scherzer and Tscharnuter,[87] emphasis is placed on promoting normalization of muscle tone and posture. Certainly movement, and hence, vestibular stimulation would be used to achieve this normalization. Although one does not have to be trained in the NDT approach to emphasize these developmental areas, the NDT curriculum does stress them. Thus, a therapist trained in NDT may be more likely to recognize and treat abnormalities in postural tone and quality of postural responses. Similarly, therapists who are trained in sensory integration are accustomed to analyzing and treating those deficits related to vestibular dysfunction. Although we requested that the therapists who provided the outside intervention refrain from using rotary vestibular stimulation, the control (and possibly treatment) group(s) may have received sensorimotor input or other forms of vestibular stimulation which was sufficient to mask the treatment effects of this study.

Both groups of children in this study may also have benefitted from home stimulation. Therapists with advanced training and those participating in organized early intervention programs have been reported to emphasize parental involvement,[88] which is also strongly advocated in the NDT approach. Parental involvement could have led to enriched home environments which stimulated the children to the point that extra vestibular input was superfluous. This explanation also would support earlier findings[89,90] that children with Down syndrome who are reared at home show signs of better motor development than those reared outside the home. The significance of parents' inclusion in early intervention programs is unquestioned.[88,91,92] Taft[92] explains the role of parents as being nature's way of assuring that the developmental process is enhanced.

If, indeed, parental involvement and subsequent stimulation were responsible for the motor gains exhibited by the subjects in this study, then another potentially important explanation is offered regarding differences between this study and that of Ottenbacher and colleagues.[48] The institutionalized subjects in the latter study may have benefitted from the additional experimental stimulation which home-reared children in the present study may have already received through family interactions. In the future investigators may want to examine the baseline level of sensory stimulation to which their treatment and control subjects are exposed.

Clearly, additional investigations are necessary in order to clarify the relationships between muscle tone, age, specific disabilities, and parameters of effective vestibular intervention. For example, the present study was similar in design to that of Kantner and colleagues,[68] but different results were obtained in this study. Potential sources of difference between the studies include the ages of subjects, and the frequency of treatment. Of the four children with Down syndrome in Kantner and colleagues' study, only one was as young as the subjects in the present study. Further, the treatment conditions for the infants in the Kantner study were laboratory-controlled, and treatment was given more frequently (five times weekly) over a shorter time period (two weeks) than in this study. Whether differential treatment effects would have been obtained with more intense stimulation than that used in this study is not known. The value of such questions need to be considered not only in light of their empirical significance but also in terms of the practicality and the clinical implications of administering frequent, intense sensory stimulation.

Some indications from this study are that the treatment children received some benefits not realized by the control children. The children in the treatment group were subjectively noted by the interveners and the examiner to have better tone and better quality of movement after 12 weeks of intervention. No children in the control group, but two children in the treatment group scored age-appropriately on the Gross Motor section of the PDMS at the end of the study. Additionally, five parents as well as interveners documented increased alertness in treatment but not in control children. The fact that other studies[52,53,93] have also reported increased alerting in a variety of children exposed to vestibular stimulation indicates that this variable may be an important one to quantify in future research and to observe clinically. Possibly other variables related to alerting are affected by vestibular stimulation but are not identified by motor assessment tools.

SUMMARY AND RECOMMENDATIONS
FOR FUTURE STUDY

Positive clinical information obtained from this study indicates that Down syndrome infants can make significant motor advancements which can be documented by both the MAI[50] and the newly revised PDMS.[51] This information is important for a number of reasons. First, it indicates that, over a 12 week period, therapists can expect to see motor changes in

Down syndrome infants. Second, this study provides relevant test data regarding two new motor assessments likely to be widely used by physical and occupational therapists.

A methodological suggestion related to demonstrating positive effects of vestibular stimulation emerges from the present study. Although efforts were made to match the children and control for extraneous intervention, nuisance variables were encountered. Since the coordinator of the project would have known the group assignment of the children, an outside examiner naive to group assignment performed all assessments. This controlled for examiner bias but decreased the contact which the coordinator had with the parents. The checklists which the parents completed at each evaluation session were invaluable in providing information about children's illnesses, attendance in outside clinical intervention, and the types of personnel providing this additional intervention. Without the checklists, these changes could have remained unknown to the coordinator, who used them to offer possible reasons for the results of the study. The use of such an instrument is highly recommended in future studies of this type.

Results of the checklists indicated that a large number of parents of treatment subjects and no parents of controls reported increased alertness in their children. Subsequent investigations should explore the effects of rotary stimulation on such measures as behavioral state, as well as social interactional variables. Alertness could serve to increase the interactions between the child with Down syndrome and persons and objects in his or her environment. In turn, increased exploration of the environment could lead to better motor development. Controlled rotary vestibular stimulation may also have a greater effect on arousal than on motor performance of infants with Down syndrome.

Investigations with larger sample sizes would help reduce the chance of committing a Type II error. Obtaining such a large sample is difficult unless one is affiliated with a clinic specifically serving children with Down syndrome. Therapists working in such clinical settings could participate in such studies which would contribute to the knowledge of the effects of sensory stimulation and motor development in different clinic populations. Clinical researchers should be familiar with the implications of small sample sizes and the uses of power analyses as recommended by Ottenbacher[94] for examining often subtle clinical treatment effects.

An equally important consideration related to sample size is that many parents of infants with Down syndrome (or other disabilities) may not be inclined to participate in research projects. Parents of infants with Down syndrome, especially those with infants under six months of age, are still undergoing adjustments. Although great strides have been made in improving the developmental achievements of these infants, Down syndrome always causes mental retardation. This fact alone requires tremendous personal and familial adjustment to which clinicians and researchers must be sensitive.

The checklist data from this study suggest that benefits may be achieved by infants with Down syndrome receiving therapy from clinicians who have specific training in NDT or sensory integration. Further investigations, designed to analyze the benefits of these two approaches are warranted. These studies should incorporate the findings of Harris[37] who, upon her inability to show significant effects of NDT intervention, attributed this to a small sample size and insensitive measuring tools. Perhaps the new data generated by this study as well as the authors' earlier work[49] regarding the MAI and the PDMS, supply the foundation for future examinations of motor assessment tools.

Despite the negative interaction effects reported in this study, the authors believe that continued investigations are needed to clarify the effects of vestibular and other forms of sensory stimulation on various types and ages of developmentally delayed populations. Future studies need to explore the effects of rotary, as well as other vestibular stimulation, such as rocking, which have affected behavioral change in premature infants who exhibit lower muscle tone than fullterm infants.[53,55,58,60,62] At present, many investigators have reported positive effects of vestibular stimulation; the negative findings of the present study and that of Sellick and Over[70] should serve not to diminish research but to help clarify the nature of subject characteristics, variables, and parameters of studies exploring the efficacy of vestibular stimulation.

REFERENCES

1. *National Research Strategy for Neurological and Communicative Disorders* NIH Publication No 79-1910. National Institute of Health, 1979.
2. Kirman B: General aspects of Down's syndrome. *Physiotherapy* 62 (1): 1-4, 1976.
3. Weeks ZR: Effects of the vestibular system on human development. Part I. Overview of functions and effects of stimulation. *Am J Occup Ther* 33(6): 376-381, 1979.
4. Coleman M: Down's syndrome. *Pediatr Ann* 7(2): 90-103, 1978.
5. Fritch U, Fritch CD: Specific motor disabilities in Down's syndrome. *J Child Psychol Psychiatry* 15: 293-301, 1974.
6. Hall B: Mongolism in newborns: A clinical and cytogenetic study. *Acta Paediatr Scand Suppl* 154, 1964.
7. Loesch-Mdzewska D: Some aspects of neurology of Down's syndrome. *J Ment Defic Res* 12: 237-246, 1968.
8. Levinson A, Friedman A, Stamps F: Variability of mongolism. *Pediatrics* 16: 43-53, 1955.
9. Kugel RB: Combating retardation in infants with Down's syndrome. *Ment Retard* 17: 188-192, 1970.
10. Kugel RB, Reque D: A comparison of mongoloid children. *J Am Med Assoc* 175: 959-961, 1961.
11. McIntire MS, Menolascino FJ, Wiley JH: Mongolism-some clinical aspects. *Am J Ment Defic* 69: 794-800, 1965.
12. Rapin I: Hypoactive labyrinths and motor development. *Clin Pediatr* 13(11): 922-936, 1974.
13. Cowie VA: *A Study of the Early Development of Mongols*. London. Pergamon Press, 1970.

14. Haley SM: *Postural reactions: Developmental and functional considerations.* Read before the Eunice Kennedy Shriver Center Conference, Boston, MA, May, 1984.

15. Harris SR: *Development of tone in the normal infant and the infant with Down syndrome.* Read before the Eunice Kennedy Shriver Center Conference, Boston, MA, May, 1984.

16. Share JB, Veale AMO: *Developmental Landmarks for Children with Down's Syndrome.* Dunedin, New Zealand, University of Otago Press, 1974.

17. Lydic JS, Steele C: Assessment of the quality of sitting and gait patterns in children with Down's syndrome. *Phys Ther* 59(12): 1489-1494, 1979.

18. Nathan D: *Development of Creeping in a Normal and a Down Syndrome Infant,* thesis. Boston University, Boston, MA, 1979.

19. Connolly B, Morgan S, Russell FF, Richardson B: Early intervention with Down syndrome children. *Phys Ther* 60(11): 1405-1408, 1980.

20. Connolly B, Russell FF: Interdisciplinary early intervention program. *Phys Ther* 56(2): 155-158, 1976.

21. Harris SR: Transdisciplinary therapy model for the infant with Down's syndrome. *Phys Ther* 60(4): 420-423, 1980.

22. Zausmer E: The evaluation of motor development in children. *Phys Ther* 44(4): 247-250, 1964.

23. Zausmer E: Early developmental stimulation, in Pueschel SM (ed): *Down Syndrome: Growing and Learning.* Kansas City, Andrews and McMeel, Inc, 1978.

24. Zausmer E: Gross motor stimulation, in Pueschel SM (ed): *Down Syndrome: Growing and Learning.* Kansas City, Andrews and McMeel, Inc, 1978.

25. Zausmer E, Peuschel SM, Shea A: A sensory motor stimulation program for the young child with Down's syndrome: A preliminary report. *MCH Exchange* 2(4): 25-29, 1971.

26. Dmitriev V: Exercises for the infant birth to six months. *Sharing Our Caring* 1(4): 25-29, 1971.

27. Dmitriev V: Teaching motor skills to Down's syndrome children in a preschool setting. *Sharing Our Caring* 1(5): 13-15, 1971.

28. Hanson M: *Teaching a Down's Syndrome Infant.* Baltimore, University Park Press, 1976.

29. Knights RM, Hyman JA, Wozny MA: Psychomotor abilities of familial, brain-injured and mongoloid retarded children. *Am J Ment Defic* 70: 454-457, 1965.

30. Levine B, Birch A: Physical and occupational therapy, in Wortis J (ed): *Mental Retardation and Developmental Disabilities.* New York, Brunner/Mazel, 1977, vol 9, pp 132-140.

31. MacLean WE, Baumeister AA: Effects of vestibular stimulation on motor development and stereotyped behavior of developmentally delayed children. *J Abn Child Psychol* 10(2): 229-245, 1981.

32. Mahoney G, Glover A, Finger I: Relationship between language and sensorimotor development of Down syndrome and nonretarded children. *Am J Ment Defic* 86(1): 21-27, 1981.

33. Pesh RD, Nagy DK, Caden BW: A survey of the visual and developmental-perceptual abilities of the Down syndrome child. *J Am Optometric Assoc* 49(9): 1031-1037, 1978.

34. Pueschel SM: *Down Syndrome: Growing and Learning.* Kansas City, Andrews and McMeel, Inc, 1981.

35. Lydic JS: Motor development in children with Down's syndrome. *Sharing Our Caring* 10(3): 3-6, 1980.

36. Lydic JS: *Characteristics of Physical and Occupational Therapy with Mentally Retarded Individuals.* Unpublished manuscript, 1983.

37. Harris SR: Effects of neurodevelopmental therapy on motor performance of infants with Down's syndrome. *Dev Med Child Neurol* 23: 477-483, 1981.

38. Bayley N: *The Bayley Scales of Infant Development.* New York, Psychological Corporation, 1969.

39. Folio M, Dubose RF: *Peabody Developmental Motor Scales.* Nashville, TN, George Peabody College for Teachers, 1974.

40. Stedman DJ, Eichorn DH: A comparison of growth and development of institutionalized and home-reared mongoloids during infancy and early childhood. *Am J Ment Defic* 69(3): 391-401, 1964.

41. Laveck B, Brehm SS: Individual variability among children with Down's syndrome. *Ment Retard* 16(2): 135-137, 1978.

42. Laveck B, Laveck G: Sex differences in development among children with Down syndrome. *J Pediatr* 91(5): 767-769, 1977.

43. Eipper D, Azen S: A comparison of two developmental instruments in evaluating children with Down's syndrome. *Phys Ther* 58(9): 1066-1069, 1979.

44. Ramsay M, Piper MC: A comparison of two developmental scales in evaluating infants with Down syndrome. *Early Hum Dev* 4(1): 89-95, 1980.

45. Harris SR: Relationship of mental and motor development in Down's syndrome infants. *Phys Occup Ther Pediatr* 1(3): 13-18, 1981.

46. Fishler, K, Share J, Koch R: Adaptation of Gesell developmental scales for evaluation of development in children with Down's syndrome. *Am J Ment Defic* 68: 642-646, 1964.

47. Dicks-Mireaux M: Mental development of infants with Down's syndrome. *Am J Ment Defic* 77(1): 26-32, 1972.

48. Ottenbacher K, Short MA, Watson PJ: The effects of a clinically applied program of vestibular stimulation on the neuromotor performance of children with severe developmental disability. *Phys Occup Ther Pediatr* 1(3): 1-11, 1981.

49. Lydic JS, Short MA, Nelson DL: Comparison of two scales for assessing motor development in infants with Down's syndrome. *Occup Ther J Res* 3(4): 213-221, 1984.

50. Chandler L, Andrews M, Swanson M: *Movement Assessment of Infants.* Rolling Bay, WA, AM Larson, 1980.

51. Folio M, Fewell R: *Peabody Developmental Motor Scales.* Hingham, MA, Teaching Resources Corporation, 1983.

52. Gregg C, Haffner M, Korner A: The relative efficacy of vestibular proprioceptive stimulation and the upright position in enhancing visual pursuits in neonates. *Child Dev* 47: 309-314, 1976.

53. Neal MV: *The Relationship Between a Regimen of Vestibular Stimulation and the Developmental Behavior of the Premature Infant,* dissertation. New York University, New York, 1967.

54. White B, Castle P: Visual exploratory behavior following postnatal handling of human infants. *Percept Motor Skills* 18: 495-502, 1964.

55. Freedman D, Boverman H: The effects of kinesthetic stimulation on certain aspects of development in premature infants. *Am J Orthopsychiatry* 36: 223-225, 1966.

56. Hasselmeyer E: The premature neonate's response to handling. *Am Nurs Assoc* 11:15-24, 1964.

57. Rice RD: Premature infants respond to sensory stimulation. *Am Psychiatry Assoc Mon:* 8-9, Nov, 1975.

58. Korner A, Thoman E: The relative efficacy of contact and vestibular-proprioceptive stimulation in soothing neonates. *Child Dev* 43: 443-453, 1972.

59. Korner A, Thoman E: Visual alertness in neonates as evoked by maternal care. *J Exp Child Psychol* 10: 67-78, 1972.

60. Pederson D, TerVrugt D: The influence of amplitude and frequency of vestibular stimulation on the activity of two-month-old infants. *Child Dev* 44:122-128, 1973.

61. Pomerleau-Malcuit A, Clifton R: Neonatal heart rate response to tactile, auditory, and vestibular stimulation in different states. *Child Dev* 44:485-496, 1980.

62. TerVrugt D, Pederson D: The effect of vertical rocking frequencies on the arousal level in two-month-old infants. *Child Dev* 44: 122-128, 1973.

63. Clark D, Kreutzberg J, Chee FKW: Vestibular stimulation influence on motor development in infants. *Science* 196: 1228-1229, 1977.

64. Kreutzberg J: *Effects of Vestibular Stimulation on the Reflex and Motor Development in Normal Infants,* thesis. The Ohio State University, Columbus, OH, 1976.

65. Solkoff N, Yaffe E, Weintraub D: Effects of handling on the subsequent development of premature infants. *Dev Psychol* 1: 765-768, 1969.

66. Chee FKW, Kreutzberg J, Clark D: Semicircular canal stimulation in cerebral palsied children. *Phys Ther* 58: 1071-1075, 1978.

67. Rogos R: *Clinically Applied Vestibular Stimulation and Motor Performance in Children with Cerebral Palsy,* thesis. The Ohio State University, Columbus, OH, 1977.

68. Kantner RM, Clark D, Allen L, Chase M: Effects of vestibular stimulation on nystagmus response and motor performance in the developmentally delayed infant. *Phys Ther* 56(4): 414-421, 1976.

69. Casler L: Supplementary auditory and vestibular stimulation: Effects on institutionalized infants. *J Exp Child Psychol* 19: 456-463, 1975.

70. Sellick K, Over R: Effects of vestibular stimulation on motor development of cerebral palsied children. *Dev Med Child Neurol* 22: 476-483, 1980.

71. Harris SR: *Reliability of the Movement Assessment of Infants.* Read before the Movement

Assessment of Infants Conference sponsored by the Massachusetts Chapter Pediatric Section of the American Physical Therapy Association, 1983.

72. Lydic JS: Motor development in children with Down syndrome. *Phys Occup Ther Pediatr* 2(4): 53-74, 1982.

73. Ottenbacher K: Developmental implications of clinically applied vestibular stimulation. *Phys Ther* 63(3): 338-342, 1982.

74. Weeks ZR: Effects of vestibular stimulation on human development. Part 2. Effects of stimulation on mentally retarded, emotionally disturbed, and learning-disabled individuals. *Am J Occup Ther* 33(7): 450-457, 1979.

75. Carr J; Mental and motor development in young mongol children. *J Ment Defic Res* 14: 205-220, 1970.

76. Griffiths MI: *Developmental Diagnosis,* ed 2. New York, Hoeber, 1941, pp 3-106.

77. Palisano RJ, Lydic JS: The Peabody Developmental Motor Scales: An analysis. *Phys Occup Ther Pediatr* 4(1): 69-75, 1984.

78. Brazelton TB: *The Neonatal Behavioral Assessment Scale.* Clinics in Developmental Medicine No 50. Philadelphia, JB Lippincott, 1973, pp 4-5.

79. Ottenbacher K: Statistical power and research in occupational therapy. *Occup Ther J Res* 2(1): 13-25, 1982.

80. Bobath B: A neuro-developmental treatment of cerebral palsy. *Physiotherapy* 49: 242-244, 1964.

81. Bobath B: The very early treatment of cerebral palsy. *Dev Med Child Neurol* 9: 373-390, 1967.

82. Ayres AJ: *Sensory Integration and Learning Disorders.* Los Angeles, Western Psychological Services, 1972, pp 113-129.

83. Ayres AJ: *The Development of Sensory Integrative Theory and Practice.* Dubuque, IA, Kendall/Hunt Publishing Co, 1974, pp 313-320.

84. Ottenbacher K: Power and non-significant research results. *Dev Med Child Neurol* 23: 663-664, 1981.

85. Campbell S: Movement Assessment of Infants: An evaluation. *Phys Occup Ther Pediatr* 1(4): 53-58, 1981.

86. Gesell A, Amatruda C: *Developmental Diagnosis,* ed 2. New York, Hoeber, 1941, pp 3-106.

87. Scherzer AL, Tscharnuter I: *Early Diagnosis and Therapy in Cerebral Palsy.* New York, Marcel Dekker, 1982.

88. Redditi JS: Occupational and physical therapy treatment components for infant intervention programs. *Phys Occup Ther Pediatr* 3(3): 33-44, 1983.

89. Centerwall SA, Centerwall WR: A study of children with mongolism reared in the home compared to those reared away from the home. *Pediatrics* 25: 678-685, 1960.

90. Donoghue C, Kirman B, Bullmore G, et al. Some factors affecting walking in a mentally retarded population. *Dev Med Child Neurol* 12: 781-792, 1970.

91. Denhoff E: A sensory motor enrichment program, in Brazelton TB, Lester B (eds): *New Approaches to Developmental Screening of Infants.* New York, Elsevier, 1983, pp 229-244.

92. Taft L: Critique of early intervention for cerebral palsy, in Brazelton TB, Lester B (eds): *New Approaches to Developmental Screening of Infants.* New York, Elsevier, 1983, pp 219-228.

93. Chee FKW: *Effects of vestibular stimulation on motor development in cerebral palsy children.* Unpublished master's thesis, the Ohio State University, Columbus, OH, 1975.

94. Ottenbacher K: The significance of power and the power of significance: Recommendations for occupational therapy research. *Occup Ther J Res* 4(1): 37-50, 1984.

A Meta-Analysis
of Applied Vestibular
Stimulation Research

Kenneth J. Ottenbacher, PhD, OTR
Paul Petersen, PhD, OTR

ABSTRACT. The results of studies examining the effectiveness of vestibular stimulation as a form of sensory stimulation were reviewed. The review employed recently developed quantitative methods that treat the literature review process as a unique type of research. Forty-one studies were located that employed some form of vestibular stimulation as the independent variable. Eighteen of these studies met criteria consistent with traditionally accepted standards of empirical inquiry in the behavioral and biomedical sciences and were included in the review. The 18 studies contained a total of 44 hypothesis tests that evaluated the efficacy of vestibular stimulation as a form of sensory enrichment designed to facilitate various developmental parameters. An analysis of the results of these tests, using methods of meta-analysis, revealed that subjects receiving vestibular stimulation performed significantly better than members of control or comparison groups who did not receive such stimulation.

INTRODUCTION

The therapeutic application of sensory enrichment experiences designed for infants at risk and young children with overt developmental delay has expanded rapidly over the past decade. Ferry recently observed that, "There has been an exponential proliferation of developmental stimulation programs for environmentally deprived children."[1(p38)] Although such programs are popular forms of therapy for the developmentally delayed pediatric population, considerable debate exists among health care providers and educators concerning their empirically demonstrated effectiveness.[2-6] Campbell recently commented on some of the possible nega-

Kenneth J. Ottenbacher is Assistant Professor of Occupational Therapy at the University of Wisconsin-Madison. Paul Petersen is Assistant Professor of Occupational Therapy at Elizabethtown College, Elizabethtown, PA.

Address all correspondence to K. Ottenbacher, 2120 Medical Sciences Center, 1300 University Avenue, Madison, WI 53706.

tive effects generated by the controversy surrounding the efficacy of early intervention.[7] She noted that additional research is clearly needed in this area and that therapists must be circumspect in applying therapeutic procedures and interpret their effectiveness in relation to the published research.

One particular area of sensory enrichment, the use of controlled vestibular stimulation, has been a particularly popular form of sensory stimulation therapy for at risk infants and young children with developmental delay. To date, several studies have been reported employing clinically applied vestibular stimulation to facilitate the developmental status of infants and children with developmental delays. Traditional narrative attempts to integrate literature related to the efficacy of sensory enrichment programs have failed to produce any clear degree of empirically-based consensus. As Cooper and Rosenthal have noted, however, "some of the confusion and contradiction we often convey about our research may not be a function of the results we found but of how we have chosen to synthesize them."[8(p447)]

Traditional narrative reviews of accumulated data based studies have been criticized as subjective and unscientific.[9-11] In discussing the inadequacies of traditional literature reviews Glass states that "A common method of integrating several studies with inconsistent findings is to carp on the design or analysis deficiencies of all but a few studies—those remaining frequently being one's own work or that of one's students and friends—and then advance the one or two "acceptable" studies as the truth of the matter."[10(p7)] The subjective and judgmental nature of traditional literature reviews is unfortunate because often these reviews of particular topic areas are instrumental in establishing or refuting the empirical legitimacy of a finding.

Recently, techniques that synthesize and integrate bodies of empirical literature have been developed and refined.[9,11,12] The procedures, referred to by Cooper[9] as quantitative reviewing and Glass and his colleagues as "meta-analysis", treat the literature review as a unique type of research and allow the investigator to compare quantitatively a number of research studies and to make consensual judgements based on the results. They also facilitate the systematic investigation of variation across studies, including differences in sampling procedures, research design characteristics, and the use of multiple types of dependent variables.[13]

Quantitative reviewing methods employing meta-analytic procedures have been employed to bring some degree of order to controversial bodies of literature in the behavioral sciences.[14-16] The purpose of this paper is to expose consumers of pediatric research literature to the techniques and procedures of quantitative reviewing and second, to use the procedures to evaluate the effectiveness of clinically applied vestibular stimulation to facilitate developmental parameters in normal infants, infants defined as high risk, and individuals with overt developmental delay.

METHODS

Potentially relevant studies were obtained through an on-line computer search of *Psychological Abstracts, Index Medicus, Dissertation Abstracts International,* and *Current Index to Journals in Education-Resources in Education (ERIC).* In addition to the computer searches, an examination of the bibliographies of retrieved studies (citation tracking) resulted in the location of additional information.

Relevance Decision Criteria. The search yielded a total of 41 non-over-lapping research report titles that were broadly construed as potentially relevant to the topic—the efficacy of vestibular stimulation as a form of sensory enrichment. The abstracts and full reports were then judged for relevance on several specific criteria. The first criterion for inclusion in the review was that a study had to investigate *the effects of controlled vestibular stimulation* as at least one of the independent variables. To qualify as vestibular stimulation the sensory stimulation activity had to involve procedures designed to stimulate vestibular receptors. Specifically, these activities included rotatory stimulation combined with impulsive starts and stops or linear or vertical accelerations or some combination of rotatory, linear, vertical, or sinusoidal oscillating movement. Studies in the literature which identified the independent variable as increased "handling" were included in the review only if the handling emphasized activities which primarily stimulated vestibular receptors. For example, a study by White and Castle[17] in which "handling" was identified as the primary independent variable was included in the review because the operational definition of handling in this particular investigation emphasized rocking the infant subjects for a period of up to ten minutes per session.

Studies that provided tactile stimulation as the primary method of intervention or "handling" were not included in the review. For instance, Solkoff and associates reported a study that involved increased "handling" to improve the "development of premature infants".[18] This study was not included because the independent variable (handling) was operationally defined as providing tactile stimulation (rubbing) to the neck, back, and arms, of the infants. Certainly all forms of clinically applied vestibular stimulation will involve a degree of tactile and proprioceptive stimulation. The decision to include only those studies that provided primarily "vestibular" stimulation represented a practical attempt to isolate vestibular stimulation as the principal independent variable.

The second criterion for inclusion in the review was related to the *type of dependent variable(s) employed* in the report. One advantage of quantitative reviewing methodology is that it permits the use of broad dependent variables. The purpose of this investigation was to evaluate the literature investigating the therapeutic effectiveness of clinically applied vestibular stimulation. Improvement or enhancement of development was broadly defined by performance on any measure that evaluated cognitive/language ability; motor/reflex functions; visual/auditory alertness; or physiological (weight gain, growth) functions. Studies employing only non-developmental dependent measures such as heart rate, blood pressure, or respiration rate were not included.

The last two criteria were related to the *study's design and method of analysis*. The study had to report a comparison between at least two groups—one that received vestibular stimulation and one that did not. In some cases when a within-subjects experimental design was used, the comparison or control group was the same as the experimental group. Some studies made comparisons between more than two groups. For example, Casler studied the effect of vestibular stimulation versus auditory stimulation versus a control condition in infants residing in an orphanage.[19] The subjects were divided into three groups, one receiving vestibular stimulation, one receiving auditory stimulation and a control condition. For purposes of quantitative analysis only data from the vestibular stimulation and control group were analyzed. The comparisons involving additional experimental groups receiving other forms of sensory stimulation were not included in the analysis of any of the reviewed studies. Thus, all of the analyzed comparisons involved a group of subjects receiving vestibular stimulation and a comparison or control group not receiving such stimulation.

Finally, the study had to report findings and results in a manner that allowed quantitative analysis. That is, the investigation had to report the results of statistical tests (t, F ratios, means, SD, df, p-levels, etc.) in sufficient detail so that the appropriate effect size measure could be computed.

Because they did not meet the above criteria, 14 of the 41 studies were eliminated after the available abstracts and titles were reviewed. Another 9 studies were eliminated for similar reasons after the full report was scrutinized. The remaining 18 studies met the previously outlined criteria and were included in the review.

Characteristics of Individual Studies. With the selection criteria for the studies defined and the general boundaries of the review determined, the next step was to identify aspects of the studies that might be related to study outcomes. These variables fell into four general categories:

1. Subject characteristics (i.e., number of subjects, mean ages, medical diagnoses, developmental level).
2. Design characteristics including: (a) whether the study design was between or within-subjects, (b) how the subjects were assigned (i.e., random, matched, etc.), (c) the amount of time each group spent receiving stimulation, (d) the type of independent variable (i.e., rotatory, linear, vertical or combined vestibular stimulation,

(e) the type of dependent measure used (i.e., cognitive/language, motor/reflex, visual/auditory ability, or physiological), and (f) whether the dependent measure was obtained with a standardized or non-standardized instrument.
3. Aspects of the study's outcome such as statistical test used, test value reported, corresponding probability level, degrees of freedom, and means and standard deviations.
4. Retrieval characteristics including the year of publication, whether published in a journal or other source, and how the study was located.

The information described above was coded for each of the individual studies and subjected to computer analysis.

Quantifying Outcomes

Effect Size Estimation. Procedures capable of uncovering systematic variation in study results have been pioneered by Glass.[10,12] Glass refers to the synthesis of quantitative outcomes across studies as "meta-analysis", which he defines as the "statistical analysis of a large collection of analyses of results from individual studies for the purpose of integrating the findings. It connotes a rigorous alternative to the casual, narrative discussions of research studies which typify our attempts to make sense of the rapidly expanding research literature."[10(p6)]

Significance testing at a pre-determined probability level is the *sine qua non* of traditional primary research, however, significance testing which compares an observed relation to the chance of no relation, becomes less informative as evidence supporting a phenomenon accumulates. The question of most interest to clinicians is not whether a treatment effect exists but how much of an effect exists. Effect size measures that are free of sample-size influence can play a vital role in determining the degree to which a treatment exerts an impact on a particular population.

The effect size measure used in this investigation was the d-index. The d-index gauges the difference between two group means in terms of their common (average) standard deviation. If $d = .3$, it means that $3/10$ of a standard deviation separates the average person in the two groups. This effect size transforms the results of any two group comparison into a common standardized metric regardless of the original measurement scales. Effect size measures are available which are appropriate for any type of research design or statistical analysis.[20] Cohen presents a detailed description of various effect size measures and tables to compute power, sample size, and significance level.[20] The d-index was selected because it is simple to compute, it is "scale free", and it is applicable to a plurality of studies investigating the effects of vestibular stimulation.

Effect sizes can be computed from t and F ratios when means and standard deviations are not reported. Friedman[21] has provided formulas and a rationale for transforming t and F values to d-indexes. In instances where t and F ratios are not reported, they may be estimated from the significance level and sample size.[12] When non-parametric statistics or percentages are reported, effect sizes can be computed using procedures described by Glass.[11,12] Hedges[22] has reported that d-indexes may be biased as the sample size becomes smaller (less than 50), so Hedges' correction factors were employed to adjust for potentially inflated effect sizes.

Cohen[20] presents several measures of distribution overlap developed to enhance the interpretability of effect size indexes. The overlap measure employed in this review, called U_3, indicates the percentage of the population with the smaller mean that is exceeded by the average person in the population with the larger mean. A table for converting d-indexes to U_3 values is presented by Cohen.[20(p22)]

RESULTS

Description of the literature. A total of 631 subjects participated in the 44 hypothesis tests found in the 18 studies that were included in the review. The subjects ranged in age from only a few days to the mid-sixties. Three hundred and forty-five of the participants were infants and toddlers without any identified handicapping conditions while 105 subjects were identified as "at risk" premature infants. The remaining 181 subjects were infants, children, and adults with overt developmental delay including cerebral palsy and mental retardation.

Some form of random assignment to groups or conditions was used in 11 of the 18 studies, while matching on selected characteristics was employed in six of the studies. One investigation involved pre-existing groups with no experimental manipulation in terms of assignment. The mean year of report appearance was 1977.

Two raters independently coded the type of independent variable and dependent measures employed in five studies in order to determine an indication of coding reliability. The separate codings revealed a 100 percent agreement for the 5 studies in terms of categorizing the independent variable (type of vestibular stimulation) and 89 percent agreement regarding categorization of the dependent variable. Stock and colleagues have demonstrated that study variables can be reliably coded provided raters are given some prior training.[23]

Effect Size Analysis. Table 1 lists the 18 studies included in the review, the mean d-index for that study, the associated U_3 value, and the number of hypotheses tests included in the study evaluating the efficacy of vestibular stimulation. Table 2 includes the individual d-index values. Each

Table 1. Average d-index and Associated U_3 Value for

All Studies Included in the Review

Authors	Year	Average d-index	U_3(%)	N*
Casler, L.	1975	.08	53.2	2
Cass, M.	1980	.47	68.0	3
Chee, F.W. et al	1978	1.74	95.9	2
Clark, D.C. et al	1977	1.28	89.9	2
Gregg, C.L. et al	1976	.52	69.8	2
Kantner, R.M. et al	1982	1.62	94.7	1
Korner, A.F. et al	1975	.35	63.7	1
Korner, A.F. et al	1970	2.24	98.8	1
Korner, A.F. et al	1972	.89	81.3	1
Levine, S.	1983	.56	71.2	2
Lydic, J.	1984	.21	58.3	2
Neal, M.V.	1968	.53	70.2	6
Ottenbacher, K. et al	1981	1.10	86.4	3
Pelletier, J. et al	1984	1.56	95.2	6
Rogos, R.	1977	.77	77.9	2
Sellick, K. et al	1980	.08	53.2	3
TerVurgt, D. et al	1973	.52	69.8	1
White, B.L. et al	1964	.20	57.9	4

*NOTE: N refers to the number of hypothesis tests used to compute the average d-index.

d-index is indicated by a combination of "stem" and "leaf". The "stem" includes the initial or beginning value for the d-index and appears in the left-hand margin of the table. The "leaf" values represent individual numbers, each of which is associated with the corresponding stem. For example, the numbers 2, 6, and 7 (leaf) to the right of 1.5 (stem) in Table 2 represent d-indexes of 1.52, 1.56, and 1.57 respectively. The stem and leaf table provides all the information of a histogram but also shows the actual values of all d-indexes. Below the stem and leaf table the minimum and maximum d-indexes are presented along with the first and third quartile (Q_1, Q_3) mean, median, and standard deviation.

The works of Glass, Cohen, and Friedman contain specific instructions concerning the calculation of d-indexes and examples of how effect sizes are translated into U_3 values.[12,20,21] The mean d-index for the 44 hypothe-

Table 2. Stem and leaf table showing individual d-indexes and descriptive information for effect sizes from reviewed studies.*

Stem	Leaf
2.0	1
1.9	
1.8	
1.7	
1.6	1
1.5	2 6 7
1.4	2 9
1.3	1
1.2	
1.1	3 7
1.0	8
.9	8
.8	2 3 9 9 9
.7	3 5
.6	6 9
.5	2 2
.4	4 5
.3	6 9
.2	2 3 5
.1	0 0 0 3 3 4
.0	2 5 5 6 8 9

Mean	.78	Maximum	2.73	Q_1	.13
SD	.68	Minimum	.02	Q_3	1.13
Median	.67	Total N	44		

*Two values, 2.73 and 2.24 are not included in the Table.

sis tests was .78 (SD = ±.68). Cohen has proposed labels for various effect sizes to describe their relative magnitude.[20] In the behavioral sciences Cohen interprets a d-index of .20 to .50 as small, .50 to .80 as medium, and greater than .80 as large.[20] The size of an effect, however, is a relative distinction based on the area of investigation, and no absolute criteria can be established to differentiate the clinical from the statistical significance of an effect size. Cooper presents an excellent analysis and discussion of the effects of significance and the significance of effects.[24]

The U_3 associated with the d-index of .78 is 78.2. This means that the average performance of subjects in experimental groups or conditions receiving some form of vestibular stimulation was better than 78.2 percent of the subjects in comparison or control groups not receiving vestibular stimulation. Figure 1 presents a graphic display of the effect size distributions for subjects receiving some form of applied vestibular stimulation and for the control or comparison subjects not receiving vestibular stimulation. The figure makes the assumption of normally distributed effect sizes for the population of studies. To the degree that this is a valid assumption, Figure 1 provides a useful heuristic device for comparing the overall performance of the treatment and comparison or control groups.

The hypothesis tests were then broken down according to the type of stimulation received. Fifteen of the hypothesis tests employed some form of rotatory vestibular stimulation as the independent variable while the remaining 29 hypothesis tests used some form or combination of linear, vertical, or sinusoidal oscillating vestibular stimulation. The mean d-index for the 15 hypothesis tests using rotatory vestibular stimulation was .88 (SD = ±.69). The U_3 for the d-index of .88 was 81.0. This U_3 value indicates that the average subject receiving rotatory vestibular stimulation scored better than 81 percent of the individuals in the control or comparison groups not receiving such stimulation. The mean d-index for the 29 hypothesis tests using linear/vertical vestibular stimulation was .73 (SD = ±.84) and the accompanying U_3 value was 76.7.

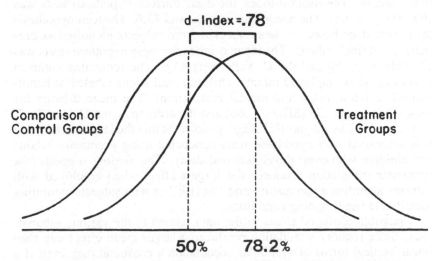

FIGURE 1. Normal curves illustrating the aggregate effect of vestibular stimulation in relation to the comparison or control groups. Data based on 44 d-indexes computed from 18 studies.

The d-indexes were next analyzed according to the type of dependent measure used to assess outcome. Twenty-five hypothesis tests employed a dependent measure of motor/reflex function. These measures included performance on standardized tests of motor ability such as the motor scale of the Bayley Scales of Infant Development as well as informal developmental measures of both gross and fine motor performance and measures of reflex function. The mean d-index for these hypothesis tests was .95 (SD = $\pm$.72) and the associated U_3 value was 82.9. Six hypothesis tests used a dependent measure that was classified as cognitive/language. These measures included scores from developmental scales as well as informal measures. The mean d-index for these hypothesis tests was .38 (SD = $\pm$.69) and the U_3 was 64.8. Seven hypothesis tests were analyzed that employed a dependent measure identified as physiological in nature. These measures included such things as judgements related to overall arousal level or growth as measured in terms of weight gain or increase in length. The mean d-index for these dependent measures was .35 (SD = $\pm$.32) and the U_3 was 63.7. Finally, six hypothesis tests were found that used a measure of visual or auditory ability (only one test measured auditory ability). The mean d-index for these tests was .94 (SD = $\pm$.68) and the U_3 was 82.6.

Following the analysis according to the type of dependent variable the effect sizes were analyzed according to diagnostic category. Thirteen hypothesis tests were conducted employing subjects identified as "normal" infants. The mean d-index for these thirteen hypothesis tests was .63 (SD = $\pm$.68). The accompanying U_3 was 73.6. Thirteen hypothesis tests were done based on data collected from subjects identified as premature "at risk" infants. The mean d-index for these hypothesis tests was .98 (SD = $\pm$.74) and the U_3 value was 83.6. The remaining eighteen hypothesis tests employed infants, children, and adults labeled as handicapped (cerebral palsy and mental retardation). The mean d-index for these 18 tests was .73 (SD = $\pm$.66) and the accompanying U_3 was 76.7.

The analysis by diagnostic category indicates that the largest effect size was associated with hypothesis tests conducted using premature infants and children with overt developmental delay. This finding suggests that vestibular stimulation produces the largest effect when employed with subjects identified as premature and "at risk" or with subjects exhibiting identifiable handicapping conditions.

A possible confound exists in the data related to the various subanalyses. Since rotatory stimulation produced a larger mean effect size than linear/vertical forms of vestibular stimulation a confound may exist if a majority of the hypothesis tests within a particular diagnostic category used rotatory vestibular stimulation as the independent variable. A similar confound may exist with the subanalyses by type of dependent measure. The dependent measures categorized as motor/reflex and visual/auditory ability were found to have relatively larger effect sizes when compared to those hypothesis tests employing dependent measures labeled as physiological or cognitive/language. If a majority of the hypothesis tests employing dependent measures of motor/reflex function or visual/auditory ability also employed rotatory rather than linear/vertical vestibular stimulation, then a confound may exist.

Inspection of the hypothesis tests by type of dependent measure revealed that for the motor/reflex dependent measures 52 percent of the hypothesis tests used rotatory vestibular stimulation. Fifty percent of the tests using a dependent measure of cognitive/language function used rotatory stimulation while none of the hypothesis tests using dependent measures labeled as physiological or visual/auditory used rotatory vestibular stimulation as the independent variable.

A similar uneven relationship was found between type of vestibular stimulation and diagnostic category, i.e., normal infants, versus premature infants or handicapped individuals. Forty-two percent of the hypothesis tests conducted with premature "at risk" infants or handicapped infants, children, and adults employed some form of rotatory vestibular stimulation as the independent variable while only fifteen percent of the hypothesis tests conducted using subjects identified as "normal" infants used rotatory vestibular stimulation as the independent variable ($X^2 = 2.85$, p $<.10$, df $= 1$).

These results suggest that a confound may exist between type of stimulation and type of dependent measure or diagnostic category. The possibility of a confound makes the results of the subanalyses more difficult to interpret. The overall d-index, however, collapsed across types of vestibular stimulation, remains unaffected by the interpretive difficulties of the subanalyses.

Finally, correlation coefficients were computed to determine if relations existed between d-indexes and other study characteristics. Correlations were computed between d-indexes and length of the study, i.e., the overall duration of vestibular stimulation (r $= .11$); between d-indexes and type of design (between versus within-subjects) (rho $= .19$), between d-indexes and type of assignment procedures (rho $= .22$); between d-indexes and whether or not the dependent measure was standardized or informal (rho $= .28$); and between d-indexes and whether or not the dependent variable was blindly recorded (rho $= .12$). All of these correlations were non-significant suggesting that these particular design characteristics were not associated with study outcome as measured by effect size.

A correlation of -.31 (p $< .05$) was found between age of the participants and d-indexes. This correlation suggests that a trend may exist in which larger effect sizes were negatively correlated with age of the subjects.

DISCUSSION

The decision to include only studies that met certain preselected criteria in the review eliminated a number of studies related to the issue under investigation. Several of these studies used some form of vestibular stimulation in conjunction with other forms of sensory enrichment such as tactile or auditory stimulation. For example, two studies, one by Kramer and Pierpont[25] and another by Barnard[26] both employed vestibular stimulation combined with auditory stimulation to enhance the development of premature infants. Both studies reported increases in growth and weight for the stimulated infants. Barnard also reported greater visual, auditory and motor maturity for the subjects of her study.[26]

Several other studies employed a combination of planned tactile stimulation and controlled vestibular stimulation. For example, Rice[27,28] developed a program of sensorimotor stimulation that involves a structured technique of cephalocaudal stroking and massage of the skin. This program consists of a specific pattern of stroking and a recommended number of massage movements for a particular body part. Following the structured tactile stimulation each infant is rocked for a specified period of time. In a study of the program Rice[28] randomly assigned thirty premature infants to experimental or control conditions. The experimental group received the Rice Infant Sensorimotor Stimulation program and the control infants received standard care for premature infants. The treatment period lasted one month. At the end of four weeks the treatment group demonstrated significantly greater weight gain and improved performance on selected postural reflexes. The treatment infants also scored significantly higher on the Bayley Mental Development Index than did the control infants. Other studies which also combined vestibular and tactile stimulation were found but not included in the analysis.[27,29-31] The sample size and design of these investigations did not allow any judgments to be made concerning the separate effects of the different types of stimulus provided during the intervention period.

The literature on early human development has frequently stressed the importance of contact and tactile stimulation as essential for normal development.[32] Korner and Thoman have postulated that the vestibular stimulation which accompanies most contact experiences, is related to the acquisition of certain developmental parameters.[33] Korner and Thoman state that "vestibular stimulation which almost invariably attends body contact and tactile stimulation appears to be a hidden form of stimulation, the importance of which is frequently overlooked".[33(p72)]

All of the studies included in the meta-analysis employed some form of vestibular stimulation as the independent variable. It is virtually impossible to functionally isolate the proprioceptive or tactile component from vestibular stimulation. The studies referred to above were not included in the review because they specifically emphasized tactile stimulation along with vestibular and other forms of sensory input. In several of the studies tactile stimulation was operationally defined as the primary independent variable. The studies included in the meta-analysis emphasized vestibular stimulation as the primary independent variable and any tactile input that was provided was incidental to the vestibular stimulation. The inclusion of studies such as that by Kramer and Pierpont,[25] Barnard[26] and others would have strengthened the outcome of the analysis, but would have introduced a possible confound with the independent variable: vestibular stimulation.

In addition to excluding studies which employed multiple types of sensory stimulation as the independent variable, several studies were located which were not included in the review because of the lack of a control or comparison group or the inability to generate an effect size from the information provided. Generally, these studies involved some type of intensive (single subject) design. For example, MacLean and Baumeister reported a study in which four developmentally delayed infants were provided rotatory vestibular stimulation.[34] Following two weeks of daily vestibular stimulation the authors reported that "all of the children showed motor and/or reflex changes that were attributable to the vestibular stimulation".[34(p229)] Kantner and associates reported a similar study in which a program of rotatory vestibular stimulation was found to produce improved motor abilities in a 6-month-old infant with Down Syndrome.[35] These "qualitative studies" add credence to the hypothesis that controlled vestibular stimulation may have a facilitory effect upon selected developmental measures in the handicapped pediatric population. The "qualitative" nature of these studies, however, did not permit them to be included in the present quantitative review.

The results of this research have quantitatively demonstrated the effect of vestibular stimulation in the studies reviewed; however, the limitations of this review should be emphasized. In spite of the popularity of therapeutic interventions promoting the use of sensory stimulation, and vestibular stimulation in particular, only eighteen studies that met the pre-established criteria for inclusion in the review were found. The criteria for inclusion in the review were specifically developed to meet empirical standards commensurate with traditional inferential research in the behavioral sciences. Clearly more studies are needed to resolve some of the questions of interpretation raised in this review.

The validity of literature review conclusions cannot be taken for granted. A reviewer performing a traditional narrative literature review makes numerous decisions bearing on the outcome of the review and each choice contains threats to the validity of the outcome.[9] Cooper and Rosenthal recently compared the use of quantitative versus traditional procedures for summarizing research findings.[8] The results demonstrated that the use of quantitative techniques increased the perceived support for, and the estimated magnitude of, the effects being reviewed. Cooper and Rosenthal note that conclusions based on meta-analysis will appear to be (and indeed they will be) more rigorous and objective than conclusions based on traditional narrative methods of integration. As noted in a previous section, Cooper and Rosenthal contend that the use of such procedures can help reduce the "contradiction" surrounding the integration and synthesis of some bodies of research literature.[8]

The procedures described in this review can help clarify and establish the clinical utility of empirical literature produced in many areas of pediatric developmental disabilities. Meta-analytic procedures provide a methodology designed to synthesize systematically a scientific information base by clarifying and defining review procedures, establishing study effect sizes in areas of research interest, and explaining how relationships of interest are modified by study variables and characteristics. Obviously, meta-analysis procedures are not a panacea. They contain aspects of both art and science, as does all research. The science is revealed in the systematic application and definition of a research methodology related to literature reviewing, while the art refers to the judgments that need to be made in the application of the procedures. Like all research methods, quantitative research reviewing involves assumptions that must be made explicit, and if these assumptions are not clear to the user or reader, misleading results and conclusions may occur.

In spite of the obvious limitations, quantitative reviewing procedures represent a significant advance over the traditional narrative method of integrating quantitative research related to the effectiveness of various forms of sensory enrichment, as well as many other areas of research in pediatric developmental disabilities.

REFERENCES

1. Ferry PC: On growing new neurons: Are early intervention programs effective. *Pediatrics* 67:38-41, 1981.

2. Denhoff E: Current status of infant stimulation or enrichment programs for children with developmental disabilities. *Pediatrics* 67:32-37, 1981.

3. Browder JA: The pediatrician's orientation to infant stimulation programs. *Pediatrics* 67: 42-45, 1981.

4. Bricker D, Carlson L, Schwarz R: A discussion of early intervention for infants with Down's Syndrome. *Pediatrics* 67:45-52, 1981.

5. Rutter M: The long-term effects of early experience. *Dev Med Child Neurol* 22:800-827, 1980.

6. Pearson P: The results of treatment: The horns of our dilemma. (Editorial) *Dev Med Child Neurol* 24:417-418, 1982.

7. Campbell S: Editorial. *Phys Occup Ther Pediatr* 2(2/3): 1-2, 1982.

8. Cooper HM, Rosenthal R: Statistical versus traditional procedures for summarizing research findings. *Psychol Bull* 87:442-449, 1980.

9. Cooper HM: Scientific guidelines for conducting integrative research reviews. *Rev Educ Res* 52:291-301, 1982.

10. Glass GV: Primary, secondary and meta-analysis of research. *Educ Res* 5:3-9, 1976.

11. Glass GV, McGaw B, Smith ML: *Meta-Analysis in Social Research.* Beverly Hills, CA, Sage, 1981.

12. Glass GV: Integrating findings: The meta-analysis of research, in *Review of Research in Education,* vol 5. Itasca, IL, FE Peacock, 1977.
13. Pillemer DB, Light RJ: Synthesizing outcomes: How to use research from many studies. *Harvard Educ Rev* 50:176-189, 1980.
14. Kavale K: The relationship between auditory perceptual skills and reading ability: A meta-analysis. *J Learn Disabil* 14:539-546, 1981.
15. Ottenbacher K: Sensory integrative therapy: Affect or effect. *Am J Occup Ther* 36:571-578, 1982.
16. Ottenbacher K, Cooper HM: Drug treatments of hyperactivity. *Dev Med Child Neurol* 25: 358-366, 1983.
17. White B, Castle P: Visual exploratory behavior following postnatal handling of human infants. *Percept Mot Skill* 18:495-501, 1964.
18. Solokoff N, Yaffe E, Weintraub D, Blase B: Effects of handling on the subsequent development of premature infants. *Dev Psychol* 11:755-761, 1969.
19. Casler L: Supplementary auditory and vestibular stimulation: Effects on institutionalized infants. *J Exp Child Psychol* 19:456-469, 1975.
20. Cohen J: *Statistical Power Analysis for the Behavioral Sciences,* revised ed. New York, Academic Press, 1977.
21. Friedman, H: Magnitude of experimental effect and a table for its estimation. *Psychol Bull* 70:245-251, 1968.
22. Hedges L: Unbiased estimation of effect size. *Eval Educ* 4:25-34, 1980.
23. Stock WA, Okan A, Haring MJ et al.: Rigor in data synthesis: A case study of reliability in meta-analysis. *Educ Res* 11:10-18, 1982.
24. Cooper HM: On the significance of effects and the effects of significance. *J Personal Soc Psych* 41:1013-1026, 1981.
25. Kramer LI, Pierpont ME: Rocking waterbeds and auditory stimuli to enhance growth of preterm infants. *J Pediatr* 88:297-309, 1976.
26. Barnard KE: *The Effect of Stimulation on the Duration and Amount of Sleep and Wakefulness in the Premature Infant.* Ann Arbor, MI, University Microfilms, 1972.
27. Rice RD: Neurophysiological development in premature infants following stimulation. *Dev Psychol* 13:69-76, 1977.
28. Rice RD: The effects of the Rice Infant Sensorimotor Stimulation treatment on the development of high-risk infants. *Birth Defects: Original Article Series* 15:7-26, 1979.
29. Powell LF: The effect of extra stimulation and maternal involvement on the development of low birth-weight infants and on maternal behavior. *Child Dev* 45:106-113, 1974.
30. Rose SA, Schmidt K, Riese ML, Bridger WL: Effects of prematurity and early intervention on responsivity to tactual stimulation: A comparison of preterm and full-term infants. *Child Dev* 51: 416-425, 1980.
31. Scarr-Salapatek S, Williams ML: The effects of early stimulation on low-birth-weight infants. *Child Dev* 44:94-101, 1973.
32. Mason WA: Early social deprivation in the non-human primates: Implications for human behavior in environmental influences, in Glass DC (ed): *Environmental Influences.* New York, Rockefeller University Press & Russell Sage Foundation, 1968, p 70.
33. Korner AF, Thoman EB: Visual alertness in neonates as evoked by maternal care. *J Exp Child Psychol* 10:67-76, 1970.
34. MacLean WE, Baumeister AA: Effects of vestibular stimulation on motor development and stereotyped behavior of developmentally delayed children. *J Abnorm Child Psychol* 10:229-234, 1982.
35. Kantner RM, Clark DL, Allen LC, Chase M: Effects of vestibular stimulation on nystagmus response and motor performance in the developmentally delayed infant. *Phys Ther* 56:414-421, 1976.

REFERENCES: STUDIES INCLUDED IN TABLE 1

Casler L: Supplementary auditory and vestibular stimulation: Effects on institutionalized infants. *J Exp Child Psychol* 19:456-463, 1975.
Cass M: *The Effects of Vestibular Stimulation on the Sensorimotor Performance of Profoundly Retarded Individuals,* doctoral dissertation. University of Alabama, Birmingham, AL, 1980.

Chee FW, Kreutzberg JR, Clark DL. Semicircular canal stimulation in cerebral palsied children. *Phys Ther* 9:1071-1075, 1978.

Clark DL, Kreutzberg JR, Chee FW. Vestibular stimulation influence on motor development in infants. *Science* 196:1228-1229, 1977.

Gregg CL, Haffner ME, Korner AF. The relative efficacy of vestibular-proprioceptive stimulation and the upright position in enhancing visual pursuit in neonates. *Child Dev* 47:309-314, 1976.

Kantner RM, Kantner B, Clark DL. Vestibular stimulation effect on language development in mentally retarded children. *Am J Occup Ther* 36:36-41, 1982.

Korner AF, Kramer HC, Haffner ME, Cosper LM. Effects of waterbed flotation on premature infants: A pilot study. *Pediatrics* 56:361-367, 1975.

Korner AF, Thoman EB. Visual alertness in neonates as evoked by maternal care. *J Exp Child Psychol* 10:67-78, 1970.

Korner AF, Thoman EB. The relative efficacy of contact and vestibular proprioceptive stimulation in soothing neonates. *Child Dev* 43:443-453, 1972.

Levine S: *An Investigation of the Effects of Vestibular Stimulation on Object Permanence in Infants with Sensorimotor Dysfunction,* doctoral dissertation. Loyola University of Chicago, Chicago, IL, 1983.

Lydic J: *The Effect of Vestibular Stimulation on the Motor Performance of Infants with Down Syndrome,* doctoral dissertation. Boston University, Boston, MA, 1984.

Neal MV. Vestibular stimulation and developmental behavior of the small premature infant. *Nurs Res* 3:1-5, 1968.

Ottenbacher K, Short MA, Watson PJ. The effect of a clinically applied program of vestibular stimulation on the neuromotor performance of children with severe developmental delay. *Phys Occup Ther Pediatr* 1(3): 1-11, 1981.

Pelletier JM, Short MA, Nelson DL: Immediate effects of waterbed flotation on approach and avoidance behaviors of premature infants. *Phys Occup Ther Pediatr* 5(2/3):81-92, 1985.

Rogos R: *Clinically Applied Vestibular Stimulation and Motor Performance in Children with Cerebral Palsy,* thesis. Ohio State University, Columbus, OH, 1977.

Sellick KJ, Over R. Effects of vestibular stimulation on motor development of cerebral palsied children. *Dev Med Child Neurol* 22:476-483, 1980.

TerVurgt D, Pederson DR. The effects of vertical rocking frequencies on the arousal level in 2 month old infants. *Child Dev* 44:205-209, 1973.

White BL, Castle PW. Visual exploratory behavior following postnatal handling of human infants. *Percept Mot Skill* 18:497-502, 1964.

Vestibular Stimulation
as Early Experience:
Historical Perspectives
and Research Implications

Margaret A. Short, PhD, OTR

ABSTRACT. Over the past several decades, researchers in many areas in the field of early experience have changed their conclusions regarding the developmental effects of sensory stimulation. Infants are no longer viewed as passive recipients of stimulation but as active organizers, not only reacting to but also altering their environments. Researchers from the fields of maternal deprivation, environmental enrichment and specific sensory stimulation concur that environmental stimulation can effect changes in developing (and in mature) organisms. The degree of change depends upon the subjects (or clients) interaction with the stimulation. These revised conclusions bring new research approaches that acknowledge transactions between infants, clients, or research subjects and their environments. While reductionistic strategies are still necessary for isolating specific variables, ecological and transactional models are increasingly used for interpreting the effects of experimental or clinical change. The study of vestibular stimulation, in particular, should be responsive to these changes because it bridges both clinical and empirical investigations in the field of early experience. Examples of changes that may occur in the field of vestibular stimulation are: increasing use of multivariate statistical analyses; adoption of experimental methods which account for transactions between subjects and their environments; increasingly detailed descriptions about the nature, parameters and contexts of stimulation; clinical approaches that elicit and evaluate client feedback, participation, and interactions with the therapist as well as the family and home environments; increasing challenges and public debate regarding the efficacy of vestibular stimulation; and evaluations of the most effective and efficient contexts for delivering and maintaining sensorimotor therapies.

INTRODUCTION

The field of early experience is based on overlapping empirical and clinical research areas. Investigators in the empirical areas have typically examined the various effects of early stimulation and deprivation, been

Margaret A. Short is in private practice in Saratoga Springs, New York. Address all correspondence to: M. A. Short, 6 Birch Street, Saratoga Springs, NY 12866.

comparative in approach, and used as subjects different animal species, including humans. Examples of topics explored in empirical areas include: maternal deprivation, malnutrition, environmental enrichment, perceptual deprivation, and early learning. Traditionally, individuals working in this field have been experiment-oriented researchers such as psychologists, neurobiologists, or animal behaviorists whose research aims are systematic in nature, i.e., testing theories or manipulating variables in order to isolate most effective parameters. The results of studies from such empirical investigations may or may not be applied to human behavior. For example, in regard to studies of cognition, Denenberg points out that: "Animal researchers also have shown interest in the development of cognitive processes. This interest has not stemmed from a philosophy of education or an attempt to develop better methods of rearing or educating children. Instead, the basic motivation has been to find out how the brain develops and how this development is affected by various sorts of early experiences."[1(p312)]

Clinical researchers in the field of early experience more often examine human beings in either normal or clinical populations, in efficacy studies or applied investigations, comprising the areas of infant stimulation or early intervention. Within the latter category, intervention can be varied, e.g., medical, educational, family-oriented, or multidisciplinary.

The study of the effects of vestibular stimulation is particularly unique in the field of early experience because it bridges both experimental and clinical fields. For example, Clark's laboratory[2-4] has produced studies with rigorous experimental methodologies testing the effects of vestibular stimulation as a clinical strategy posed by Rood[5] and the Bobaths[6] in the 1950's and 1960's, respectively. From a different perspective, Korner and Thoman[7,8] experimented with animal and human infants and cited perceptual deprivation literature as a basis for their work. Korner and associates have subsequently produced a number of very significant clinically-relevant investigations of the effects of waterbed flotation on premature human infants.[9-11]

Vestibular stimulation is only one of many areas of perceptual or sensory stimulation, and current knowledge regarding this general field comes from such research areas as: maternal deprivation, environmental enrichment, and specific sensory stimulation. Examining each of these topics will illuminate our understanding of vestibular stimulation, as a research topic as well as a clinical intervention.

MATERNAL DEPRIVATION RESEARCH

The effects of maternal deprivation have been investigated by researchers with diverse backgrounds; yet surprisingly, similar conclusions have been reached. These conclusions have emphasized the significance of the mother as a basis of security which promotes social-emotional development as well as exploration of the environment. Exploration, in turn, leads to expanded perceptual and motor stimulation. Disruption of attachment, in the form of maternal deprivation, was believed to result in social, physical, and intellectual retardation of the deprived infant.[12-15]

Some of the most significant contributors to research in maternal deprivation were Harlow and his associates. Their original comparative studies of learning theory[16-18] led, in the 1960's, to a series of investigations of the effects of total isolation or of maternal surrogates on the development of infant rhesus monkeys.[19-21] At the same time Bowlby,[13,22] a psychoanalytic theorist, was examining the effects of institutionalization (and consequent maternal deprivation) on human infants. Also during the early 1960's, parallels were drawn between the processes of attachment and imprinting.[15,23] Ethological studies of imprinting demonstrated that some species of immature birds will, during a circumscribed period after hatching, follow whatever moves in their environment. Typically what moves is most often a parent or sibling, thus insuring protection and subsequent socialization of the immature bird with other members of its same species. In the absence of a parent, however, an immature bird will follow a variety of stimuli, depending on the conspicuousness of the stimuli and specific time intervals when the bird is particularly sensitive to imprinting.[24,25]

The similarities between the processes of human attachment and imprinting included speculations of critical periods for imprinting in birds as well as for learning, infant stimulation, and the formation of social relationships in humans.[26] Both imprinting and attachment were seen as providing bases for perceptual development;[27] and Bowlby's condition of proximity-seeking or proximity-promotion in attachment cannot be behaviorally differentiated from that of following behavior in imprinting.[15]

In the 1960's, from divergent lines of research, both Harlow[28,29] and Bowlby[13] had concluded that a mother is essential for normal infant development and that maternal deprivation can result in severe social, and other forms of, retardation. Both researchers also acknowledged the importance of a critical period during which time the infant required exposure to a consistent mother or caretaker. Research from Harlow's laboratory concurred with the conclusions drawn by psychoanalytic theory. "The results of this investigation appear to be in general accord with expectations based upon the human separation syndrome described by Bowlby"[20(p130)] and Bowlby's theory included tenets from ethological theory.[15] Thus, for a brief period there was a marriage of learning, psychoanalytic and ethological theories, all emphasizing the impact of maternal caretaking during a sensitive period of human infant development. Such widely-accepted conclusions resist change.

In 1968, Casler[30] pointed out that maternal deprivation and some instances of institutionalization coincide with reduced handling, reduced opportunities for exploration, and overall diminished stimulation. He and others concluded that institutionalization and maternal deprivation were not necessarily deleterious. Many instances of normal development were reported in infants and children separated from their own mothers and raised in institutions, isolated, adopted, raised in communal environments with multiple caretakers, or raised with peers.[31-34] The term maternal deprivation, "is misleading in that it appears that in most cases the deleterious influences are not specifically tied to the mother and are not due to deprivation."[35(p123)]

Casler negated several important issues which were widely accepted at the time. He claimed that, "the human organism does not need maternal love in order to function normally"[30(p612)] and he also pointed out that institutionalization itself was not damaging to the child. In fact, "It may even be true that institutional rearing is, in some important respects, preferable to family rearing."[30(p613)] Third, Casler claimed that the damage to infant development reported by previous maternal deprivation/institutionalization studies was, in fact, the result of insufficient perceptual stimulation.[30]

In the 1970's, research from Harlow's laboratory was revised, and in this last decade, significant changes have occurred regarding perspectives of infant development. A series of studies by Harlow and his colleagues[36-39] and by others[40] in the field illustrated that peer interaction could prevent or correct the retardation that resulted from maternal deprivation. For example, Anderson and Mason reported that "Our findings of group differences in the complexity of social organization . . . reveal an important level of social competence which cannot be seen in dyadic encounters and one that has been disregarded in previous rearing studies."[40(p689)] "There is convincing evidence that the social behavior of an individual within such a group is influenced by a broad social context, which includes other monkeys in proximity to him, their ongoing activities, and their historical and immediate relations to each other, to him and to the animal that may provide the primary occasion for his response."[40(p681)] Conclusions centered on the observation that socialization such as interaction with peers, provided sufficient perceptual stimulation to negate previous effects of what had been termed "maternal deprivation". Thus, Casler's earlier proposals were supported.

ENVIRONMENTAL ENRICHMENT AND PERCEPTUAL STIMULATION RESEARCH

A separate but related line of research into perceptual stimulation originated in the 1950's with Hebb.[41] Based on studies exploring environmental enrichment effects on rat development, Hebb concluded that perceptual stimulation enhanced development, with the greatest gains achieved when the organism was stimulated early in life. Large numbers of investigators in the fields of perceptual stimulation and deprivation explored this issue.[1] Their studies started with crude but informative studies of primate visual deprivation by Reisen[42] and continued with many sophisticated neurophysiological studies of cats.[43-45] Most of the research in sensory stimulation had been conducted with immature animals, as it was generally accepted, based on Hebb's hypotheses and other notions regarding brain development, that the immature brain was most susceptible to change. "The importance of early experience is that this is a time when organizational processes are proceeding most rapidly and hence can be modified most readily."[46(p148)] Diverse behavioral and neurophysiological effects of early sensory stimulation were reported,[47-51] and even stressful or noxious stimuli were reported to effect developmental changes in immature organisms.[52]

The current conclusion is that the environmental stimulation producing the greatest developmental impact is that which actively engages the organism in a reciprocating interchange. In regard to visual adjustments, Held reported that: "movement alone, in the absence of the opportunity for recognition of error, does not suffice to produce adaptation; it must be self-produced movement."[53(p76)] Similarly, Rosenzweig and his colleagues experimentally demonstrated that, "Mere exposure to an enriched environment does not suffice to produce cerebral effects; direct and active participation is required.[48(p46)] Walsh and Cummins concluded that, "It is apparent that subjects must interact physically with the stimuli and it seems that reafferent stimulation may be particularly important."[51(p189)] "Reafference," Held defines as, "neural excitation following sensory stimulation that is systematically dependent on movements initiated by the sensing animal."[53(p74)]

Research in the field of maternal deprivation arrived at parallel conclusions. This field shifted from exploring the negative consequences of deprivation and institutionalization to isolating and clarifying the positive aspects of attachment, or bonding. Early studies in the 1950's had emphasized the role of the mother and tended to regard the infant as a passive recipient of environmental stimulation, but the 1970's and 1980's led to a more widespread acknowledgement of the need for mutuality in bonding, of parent-infant bonding, and of the responsibilities for active roles played not just by the mother but also by the infant and infant's family. The significance of active reciprocal exchange between the infant and both parents was emphasized, with active exchange recognized as promoting more enduring consequences.[54,55] This was consistent with the conclusions from Harlow's laboratory regarding effective rehabilitation for previously deprived monkeys: "stimulation by an active, reciprocating social agent."[56(p76)] Reciprocal interchange was recognized as providing the greatest opportunity for participation in a variety of perceptually stimulating and socially meaningful activities—stimulation the significance of which Casler[30] had already identified.

CLINICAL SENSORY STIMULATION

Thus, empirical literature in early experience demonstrated that perceptual stimulation enhanced, whereas perceptual deprivation retarded, development. It made sense, then, that sensory stimulation could be useful clinically for individuals who, by genetic, biological, or environmental circumstances either exhibited developmental delays or were prevented from normal sensory/social interactions. Likewise, premature infants or infants with movement or perceptual disorders could be regarded as potentially deficient in their abilities to react to parental attempts at interaction, thus interfering with the reciprocal exchange essential for bonding. Casler had reported that, "during the early months of life, social stimulation is probably nothing more than perceptual stimulation."[30(p612)]

In the 1950's and 1960's, therapists using clinical interventions developed by Rood and the Bobaths were already using sensory stimulation to promote neuromotor development of children with sensory and motor problems.[57] Currently, sensorimotor programs are popular forms of intervention for diverse clinic populations.[58-60] Ayres' sensory integration therapy[58] focuses on vestibular and tactile stimulation, and the theoretical bases of her work derive from animal studies of environmental enrichment and sensory deprivation.[61] Ayres[58] describes some learning disabled children as perceptually deprived and emphasizes the significance of critical periods for sensory stimulation. Multimodal therapeutic stimulation has been suggested for some forms of brain damage[51] and Prescott[62] has noted the significance of "near" as opposed to "distant" sensory receptors. He states that, "The somatosensory system (cutaneous, visceral, proprioceptive and vestibular afferents) is the sensory modality that mediates the abnormalities consequent to isolation rearing; and that deprivation to the other sensory modalities during the formative periods of development will not lead to abnormal social-emotional behaviors provided somatosensory stimulation is present."[62(p67)]

THE GROWING EMPHASIS ON VESTIBULAR AND TACTILE STIMULATION

Vestibular-proprioceptive and cutaneous systems were singled out as particularly responsive in human infants. Part of this focus was related to neuroanatomical evidence indicating the pervasive interconnections between (and implied influence of these systems on) other sensory and motor systems. Another reason for this focus was the reported early maturation of tactile and vestibular-proprioceptive systems.[58,63] Korner and Thoman[8] reported that, "perhaps the reason why vestibular proprioceptive stimulation is such an adequate soother for the newborn lies in the fact that the vestibular component of this stimulation, at least, is transmitted by a highly mature system which functions well long before birth."[8(p450)]

Additionally, empirical studies had recognized the significance of contact and vestibular stimulation in parent-infant interaction. Contact comfort was an important element of both Harlow's maternal deprivation studies[64] as well as psychoanalytic interpretations of attachment.[61] Animal researchers[64,65] had demonstrated that mobile, compared to stationary, surrogate mothers, tended either to be favored by or to reduce the emotionality of infant monkeys. Similarly, they posed that, during caretaking, the process of being picked up provides vestibular stimulation which facilitates eye opening, alerting, eye scanning and even possibly promotes schema and subsequent cognitive development.[66,67]

In the 1950's and 1960's, handling was found effective in reducing stress and enhancing exploratory behavior of immature organisms.[1(ch11),52] Subsequent studies in the 1960's and 1970's examined similar effects on premature human infants. Positive effects were obtained with vestibular stimulation or rocking, or stroking premature or low birthweight infants,[68-71] however, in most of these cases, movement could not be clearly differentiated from touch, and vestibular stimulation was recognized as only one component of multisensory stimulation that was often vestibular, proprioceptive, tactile, cutaneous, olfactory, thermal and kinesthetic in nature.[8]

Presently, we recognize that, "vestibular stimulation provided as supplemental environmental enrichment can enhance arousal level, visual exploratory behavior, motor development, and reflex integration in infants who are at risk and in young children with developmental delay disorders."[72(p341)] Ottenbacher reports, that 17, "of 19 studies in which some form of vestibular stimulation was used reported positive effects in at least one area of development."[72(p341)]

APPROACHES TO RESEARCH IN VESTIBULAR STIMULATION

Current investigators are attempting to either identify the nature of specific sensory variables or to isolate parameters of specific variables that produce the greatest developmental gains. For example, some groups have compared vestibular stimulation to contact or tactile-kinesthetic stimulation and have reported differing results.[8,73] Pederson and Ter Vrugt suggest, "that amplitude as well as frequency determine the effectiveness of rocking.''[74(p126)] Ottenbacher[72] suggests numerous additional studies for clarifying the effective nature of vestibular stimulation by examining: linear vs. rotatory stimulation, the optimal speed of revolutions per minute for rotatory stimulation, the significance of head control, and the effects of stimulation with specific age groups and diagnostic categories.

These suggestions represent a reductionistic approach to research, and this kind of approach is essential for delineating specific effects of isolated variables. Currently, however, a different, more expansionistic trend toward research is evident. This trend involves studying the interactive effects and the contexts of variables and is particularly important for clinical research.

> One of the major guiding principles and aims of science has been to describe phenomena in terms of the smallest feasible number of explainer variables or mechanisms. Therefore typical experimental and conceptual approaches usually consider only the major independent variables and ignore others. There is also a strong tendency towards breaking structures down into their constituents.

> However, such an approach, though perhaps useful as an initial step, may be fundamentally inappropriate. With increased sophistication and sensitivity there arises a greater recognition of the need to take into consideration increasing numbers of contributing independent variables, and increasing numbers and complexity of interconnections and interactive effects.[75(p148)]

> The recognition of this interaction leads naturally to an ecological approach. Recent developments in physics, and the emergence of new fields such as developmental psychobiology, sensory deprivation, general systems theory, and various branches of ecology, all point to the increasing recognition of the importance of adopting a holistic perspective which includes the context within which an object is studied.[75(p2)]

ECOLOGICAL AND TRANSACTIONAL APPROACHES TO RESEARCH AND INTERVENTION

This emphasis on context is reflected in recent conclusions drawn from research in early experience. After several decades, conclusions from maternal deprivation, institutionalization, environmental enrichment, perceptual stimulation, and infant learning, have been revised. Prior to 1960, human infants were viewed as passive recipients of sensory and social stimulation, and the period of infancy was regarded as guided by maturational, more so than environmental, forces.[1(p195)] By the 1970's and

1980's, research into infant learning and perception[76-79] indicated that human infants possessed sophisticated abilities to learn, perceive, and actively manipulate their physical and social environments. Goldberg states that, "In the last fifteen years, the study of infant development has shown that the young infant is by no means passive, inert, or helpless when we consider the environment for which he or she is adapted—that is, an environment which includes a responsive caregiver . . . The sensory systems of the human infant are well developed at birth, and their initial perceptual capacities are well matched to the kind of stimulation that adults normally present to them."[56(p214)]

The infant is now credited with much greater abilities as well as responsibilities for bonding, perception—all areas of development. Further, the emphasis on critical periods has diminished. Counter to Hebb's[41] original claim in the 1950's, perceptual stimulation is now recognized as effecting changes in mature as well as immature brains. Rosenzweig[48] reported that, no critical period exists for environmental enrichment, and other research with adult and geriatric organisms support this claim.[50,75,80]

Current analyses of infant intervention research are moving away from an emphasis on early experiences and recognizing adaptability throughout the entire developmental continuum.[81,82] Horowitz[83] reminds us that human development, from birth to death, is a complex phenomenon, and, "that only a healthy respect for how complex it is will permit us to adopt a long-term strategy for unraveling the processes. . . . It has been observed that development is not a disease to be declared present or absent but a process in which the functional variables are probably changing over time."[83(p246)]

Bronfenbrenner,[84] in his examinations of remediative pre-school programs begun in the 1960's, concluded that the programs producing the greatest impact were those which considered the ecology of the participating children. Ecological intervention emphasized the provision of basic requirements for life in order to sustain the family's ability to function as a child-rearing system. Bronfenbrenner stressed that early intervention programs must take into consideration the child's family and the family's medical, economic, health, and social needs. From his examination of clinical early intervention programs, Soboloff concluded that, "early intervention results in better mobility and a better acceptance of the children when a team approach is used and the parents and siblings are involved."[85(p265)]

Animal researchers also began to emphasize multiple, social influences on infant development. Despite the original emphasis on the maternal affectional system, research from Harlow's laboratory led to investigations regarding paternal and peer influences on infant development. "It is our opinion that . . . most important from the view of the whole life-span, is agemate love, which develops first through curiosity and exploration and later through multiple forms of play.''[86(p281)] Walsh reports that, ''Even in that archetype of stimulus-response paradigms, behavioral modification, there have recently emerged more complex models of reciprocal determinism.''[75(p148)]

Clinical nursing, psychological, and early intervention researchers began emphasizing methods for enhancing parent-infant or mother-infant interactions,[87-92] and the significance of fathers, siblings and peers has been recognized in effective treatment programs.[54,85,93,94] The result is an emphasis on transactional models of treatment which acknowledge that the child and environment continuously interact upon and produce changes in each other.[95]

What do these conclusions suggest for the future of research into the effects of vestibular stimulation? Different ways of viewing research exist, and each of these must be addressed. They are: empirical, clinical, statistical, social, and ultimately ethical and political.

We can easily make predictions about empirical areas because we can benefit from prior analyses of 50 years of research in the field of early experience.[96,97] Henderson[97] points out that slow progress has been made in research that has: (1) assumed continuity between sensorimotor processes and mediating mechanisms in different species, (2) administered a global treatment that is likely to manifest many outcomes, (3) used dependent variables that may be convenient but not valid, (4) formulated experiments ''with limited theoretical or empirical foundations'', and (5) overinterpreted results.

The greatest gains in early experience research have been made by studies with: clear, logical rationales for their early manipulation and subsequent dependent variables; precisely defined stimuli; and dependent variables with inherent construct validity.[97] Senf[98] has suggested that outcome studies need to: ''(1) attend more closely to the measurement concerns surrounding both the intervention and outcome variables, (2) utilize multiple measurement of the treatment and outcome variables, and (3) utilize multivariate designs so that the study will yield greater and more meaningful information.''[98(p358)]

THE FUTURE OF VESTIBULAR STIMULATION RESEARCH

These suggestions are useful for directing future investigations into the effects of vestibular stimulation. Perhaps, however, empirical and clinical investigations should proceed in different directions. Empirical research, reductionistic in nature, does not lend itself well to transactional models, and, ''by and large developmental research has used linear rather than interactive or transactional models.''[99(p2)] Empirical research is important, not only for isolating variables, but also for generating and testing theory. For the experimentalist, it may be sufficient to manipulate variables, one at a time, in a series of studies, in order to explore quantitative and qualitative changes. In experimental fields, it is widely accepted that one study is not conclusive. Research is based on the concept of replication, of eliminating bias, identifying extraneous variables, and continually reducing variables so as to confirm or deny hypotheses. For clinical relevance, however, these small manipulations, though essential when they are accumulated, may not be meaningful individually.

Enormous changes have occurred in our understanding of human development in the last decade, and it is important that clinical and empirical research reflect that knowledge. As this review illustrates, multiple lines of research have all reached the same conclusion: the context of sensory stimulation is essential. Passive stimulation of clients, while experimentally useful, may no longer be considered the most effective form of intervention. As ecological factors are increasingly recognized, therapeutic environments are being evaluated for their overall effects on client and family responses. An example of this is the current multidisciplinary concern regarding the deleterious nature of neonatal intensive care units that not only disrupt family-infant interchange but also provide exposure of premature or ill infants to potentially damaging, repetitious, non-rhythmic, non-social stimulation.[54,100-102]

In her review of research of tactile and kinesthetic stimulation with premature infants, Ross[103] concludes: "Beyond the determination of the most effective person to intervene, researchers should assess the effects of intervention on the parents and home environments of premature infants. While positive effects from early maternal involvement in intervention have been demonstrated, the critical importance of the parent or caretaker as the primary person of intervention has not been established . . . Despite this lack of research support, it seems essential to include the parent in any intervention protocol because the eventual total care of the infant will be taken over by the parent."[103(p45)]

In a naturalistic context, vestibular stimulation of infants occurs often during caretaking, parent-infant, and peer interactions. In these contexts, vestibular stimulation cannot be isolated from other sensory interactions, as multi-sensory interaction is ongoing and changing. In some families, however, natural caretaking behaviors are interrupted. Many studies have already discussed the implications of interfering with parent-infant bonding when medically unstable infants are separated at birth from their families.[55,87,88,101] Families of children with sensory or motor impairments, and deprived families who do not understand basic principles of child care, may be in crisis and unable and, therefore, need to be taught how to identify and how to elicit infant adaptive responses. Beckwith[104] points out that families of infants at risk are often those who lack the resources to meet the additional demands and stress which may occur during parenting a special child. She suggests that, "supportive services, including family counseling and parent groups, must be considered necessary for the children's development.[104(p296)]

Parents can benefit from demonstrations of their infant's sophisticated capabilities,[105,106] and families of special children may particularly require demonstrations of how they can most effectively and safely interact with their handicapped children. Various forms of vestibular and tactile stimulation may be effective in eliciting infant responses as well as establishing an important context for increasing social interactions. The result will not only provide necessary stimulation to a potentially deprived child but also enhance reciprocal transactions between the child and the family.

Christophersen[107] points out that ideal pediatric research is both statistically and socially significant. He notes, however, that most research meets only one criterion—it is either statistically but not socially significant, or it is socially but not statistically significant. Regarding vestibular stimulation, a dialogue about these issues has already been initiated. Based on an examination of the effects of vestibular stimulation on the motor development of cerebral-palsied children, Sellick and Over[108] have suggested that the gains demonstrated by the children receiving vestibular stimulation are not great enough to justify its use as a clinical intervention. Conclusions such as these, Ottenbacher[109] points out, should not be based on single studies or on traditional statistical probability levels. Ottenbacher has re-analyzed Sellick and Over's conclusions[108] and has suggested methods for clinical researchers to deal with the issue of statistical significance in an area where treatment effects are often limited.[110,111] Failure to obtain traditional levels of statistical significance may not imply the clinical or social ineffectiveness of an independent variable. In regard to vestibular stimulation, both Sellick and Over and Ottenbacher agree that continued research needs to explore efficacy, generalizability and long-term effects.

Long-term studies of treatment effectiveness are important not only for assessing the generalizability of interventions but also for addressing such issues as cost-effectiveness.[112] Other examinations[113-115] of vestibular-related therapies have taken issue with its effectiveness as an intervention, pointing to the necessity of operationalizing and assessing the social significance of intervention. For example, vestibular stimulation may have impact on the developing child, and it may also be a useful tool for eliciting parent-infant interactions. The latter effect, if it enhances parental caretaking may, in turn, result in continued stimulation of the infant; thus parental involvement may be more socially significant than a therapist-administered program oriented solely to specific developmental needs of the child. Clinical research, by considering and evaluating contexts, may end up promoting continued therapy within families as well as documenting the significant social and developmental effects of intervention.

Social and educational policies may eventually be based on the results of efficacy studies, and the authors of these studies must be aware of the social implications of their work. If clinical research leans toward long-term, family-centered interventions, then ethical issues regarding interference with social and cultural aspects of families must also be addressed.[116] Clearly, the scope and responsibilities of clinical intervention research pose demanding challenges. In fact, different research methodologies and models;[83,117] new intervention approaches;[83,116] changes in institutions such as staff and hospital organizations;[101] restructuring human service agencies;[118] and possibly altering entire ideological systems[75,118] may be required to accommodate these new ecological perspectives.

Bronfenbrenner[119] has delineated specific dimensions for a broader approach to a scientific perspective regarding the ecology of human development. He points out that his purpose is, "to stimulate new, ecological directions of thought and activity in developmental research. Moreover, the aim is to expand our conceptions, not to substitute them for other, already existing and valuable approaches. Nor is there any implication that investigation at one system level is more important or logically prior to research at another. As scientists, we must work from different perspectives in different ways. A variety of approaches are needed if we are to make progress toward the ultimate goal of understanding human development in context."[119(p529)]

Thus, clinical researchers must continue to gain knowledge from a variety of sources including clinical and empirical research. Each approach may have its own respective aims and theoretical bases, and each may provide a relevant context for understanding the nature, interactive effects, and potential therapeutic applications of vestibular and other forms of sensory stimulation. As Denenberg accurately points out: "We know from the history of science that lines of thought and experimentation which develop independently may ultimately converge for the benefit of all."[1(p312)]

REFERENCES

1. Denenberg VH (ed): *The Development of Behavior.* Stamford, CT, Sinauer Associates, 1972.

2. Chee FKW, Kreutzberg JR, Clark DL: Semicircular canal stimulation in cerebral palsied children. *Phys Ther* 58:1071-1075, 1978.

3. Kantner RM, Clark DL, Allen LC et al.: Effects of vestibular stimulation on nystagmus response and motor performance in the developmentally delayed infant. *Phys Ther* 56:416-419, 1976.

4. Clark DL, Kreutzberg JR, Chee FKW: Vestibular stimulation influence on motor development in infants. *Science* 196:1228-1229, 1977.

5. Rood MS: Neurophysiological mechanisms utilized in the treatment of neuromuscular dysfunction. 2. *Am J Occup Ther* 10:220-225, 1956.

6. Bobath K, Bobath B: The facilitation of normal postural reactions and movements in the treatment of cerebral palsy. *Physiother* 50:246-251, 1964.

7. Thoman EB, Korner AF: Effects of vestibular stimulation on the behavior and development of infant rats. *Dev Psychol* 5:92-98, 1971.

8. Korner A, Thoman E: The relative efficacy of contact and vestibular-proprioceptive stimulation in soothing neonates. *Child Dev* 43:443-453, 1972.

9. Korner AF: Maternal rhythms and waterbeds: A form of intervention with premature infants, in Thoman EB (ed): *Origins of the Infant's Social Responsiveness* Hillsdale, NJ, 1979.

10. Korner AF, Guilleminault C, Van den Hoed J et al.: Reduction of sleep apnea and bradycardia in preterm infants on oscillating water beds: A controlled polygraphic study. *Pediatrics* 61: 528-533, 1978.

11. Korner AF, Ruppel EM, Rho JM: Effects of water beds on the sleep and motility of theophylline-treated preterm infants. *Pediatrics* 70:864-869, 1982.

12. Ainsworth MDS: The development of infant-mother attachment, in Caldwell BM, Ricciuti HN (eds): *Review of Child Development Research,* vol 3. Chicago, University of Chicago Press, 1973.

13. Bowlby J: *Attachment and Loss,* vol 1, *Attachment.* New York, Basic Books, 1969.

14. Harlow HF, Harlow MK: Social deprivation in monkeys, in *The Nature and Nurture of Behavior.* San Francisco, WH Freeman, 1973.

15. Rajecki DW, Lamb ME, Obmascher P: Toward a general theory of infantile attachment: A comparative review of aspects of the social bond. *Behav Brain Sci* 3:417-464, 1978.

16. Harlow HF: The development of learning in the rhesus monkey. *Am Scientist* 47:459-479, 1959.

17. Harlow HF, Harlow MK, Suomi SJ: From thought to therapy: Lessons from a primate laboratory. *Am Scientist* 59:538-549, 1971.

18. Harlow HF, Schlitz KA, Harlow MK: Effects of social isolation on the learning performance of rhesus monkeys. *Proceedings of 2nd International Congress Primatology,* Atlanta, GA, 1968, vol 1. New York, Karger, Basel, 1969, pp 178-185.

19. Harlow HF, Harlow MK, Dodsworth RO et al.: Maternal behavior of rhesus monkeys deprived of mothering and peer associations in infancy. *Proceedings of the American Philosophical Society* 110: 58-66, 1966.

20. Seay B, Hansen E, Harlow HF: Mother-infant separation in monkeys. *J Child Psychol Psychiatry* 3:123-132, 1962.

21. Harlow HF: Love in infant monkeys. *Scientific American* 200:68-74, 1959.

22. Bowlby J: *Maternal Care and Mental Health.* Geneva, World Health Organization, 1951.

23. Hess EH: Two conditions limiting critical age for imprinting. *J Comp Physiol Psychol* 52: 515-518, 1959.

24. Lorenz KZ: The companion in the bird's world. *Auk* 54:245-273, 1937.

25. Hinde RA: *Animal Behaviour. A Synthesis of Ethology and Comparative Psychology.* ed. 2. New York, McGraw-Hill, 1970.

26. Scott JP: Critical periods in behavioral development. *Science* 138:949-958, 1962.

27. Sluckin W, Salzen EA: Imprinting and perceptual learning, in Sluckin W (ed): *Early Learning and Early Experience.* Baltimore, Penguin Books, 1971.

28. Harlow HF: The primate socialization motives. *Transactions & Studies of the College of Physicians of Philadelphia* 33:224-237, 1966.

29. Seay B, Harlow HF: Maternal separation in the rhesus monkey. *J Nerv Ment Dis* 140:434-441, 1965.

30. Casler L: Perceptual deprivation in institutional settings, in Newton G, Levine S (eds): *Early Experience and Behavior.* Springfield, Charles C Thomas, 1968.

31. Bronfenbrenner U: Early deprivation in monkey and man, in Bronfenbrenner U (ed): *Influences on Human Development.* Hinsdale, IL, Dryden Press, 1972.

32. Clarke AM, Clarke ADB (eds): *Early Experience: Myth and Evidence.* New York, The Free Press, 1976.

33. Hoffman LW, Nye FI (eds): *Working Mothers.* San Francisco, Jossey Bass Publishers, 1974.

34. Yarrow LJ: Maternal deprivation: Toward an empirical and conceptual re-evaluation. *Psychol Bull* 58:459-90, 1961.

35. Rutter M: *Maternal Deprivation. Reassessed.* Baltimore, Penguin Books, 1972.

36. Harlow HF, Suomi SJ: Social recovery by isolation-reared monkeys. *Proc Nat Acad Sci* 68:1534-1538, 1971.

37. Novak MA, Harlow HF: Social recovery of monkeys isolated for the first year of life. 1. Rehabilitation and therapy. *Dev Psychol* 11:453-465, 1975.

38. Suomi SJ, Harlow HF: Social rehabilitation of isolate-reared monkeys. *Dev Psychol* 6: 487-496, 1972.

39. Suomi SJ, Harlow HF, Domewk CJ: Effect of repetitive infant-infant separation of young monkeys. *J Abn Psychol* 76:161-172, 1970.

40. Anderson CO, Mason WA: Early experience and complexity of social organization in groups of young rhesus monkeys (Macaca Mulatta). *J Comp Physiol Psychol* 87:681-690, 1974.

41. Hebb DO: *The Organization of Behavior.* New York, Wiley, 1949.

42. Reisen AH: Arrested vision, in *The Nature and Nurture of Behavior. Developmental Psychobiology.* San Francisco, WH Freeman, 1973.

43. Hubel DH, Wiesel TN: The period of susceptibility to the physiological effects of unilateral eye closure in kittens. *J Physiol* 206:419-436, 1970.

44. Hubel DH, Wiesel TN: Receptive fields of cells in striate cortex of very young visually inexperienced kittens. *J Neurol* 26:994-1002, 1963.

45. Blakemore C, Cooper GF: Development of the brain depends on the visual environment. *Nature* 228:477-478, 1970.

46. Scott JP: Early development, in Sluckin W (ed): *Early Learning and Early Experience.* Baltimore, Penguin Books, 1971.

47. Greenough WT: Enduring brain effects of differential experience and training, in Rosenzweig MR, Bennett EL (eds): *Neural Mechanisms of Learning and Memory.* Cambridge, MA, MIT Press, 1976.

48. Rosenzweig MR: Effects of environment on brain and behavior in animals, in Schapler E. Reichler RJ (eds): *Psychopathology and Child Development.* New York, Plenum, 1973.

49. Rosenzweig MR, Bennett EL, Diamond MC: Brain changes in response to experience, in *The Nature and Nurture of Behavior. Developmental Psychobiology.* San Francisco, WH Freeman, 1973.

50. Walsh RN, Cummins RA: Neural responses to therapeutic environments, in Walsh RN, Greenough WT (eds): *Environments as Therapy for Brain Dysfunction.* New York, Plenum, 1976.

51. Levine S: Stimulation in infancy, in *The Nature and Nurture of Behavior. Developmental Psychobiology.* San Francisco, WH Freeman, 1973.

52. Held R: Plasticity in sensory-motor systems, in *The Nature and Nurture of Behavior. Developmental Psychobiology.* San Francisco, WH Freeman, 1973.

53. Ferchmin PA, Bennett EL, Rosenzweig MR: Direct contact with enriched environment is required to alter cerebral weights in rats. *J Comp Physiol Psychol* 88:360-367, 1975.

54. Klaus MH, Kennell JH: *Parent-Infant Bonding,* ed 2. St. Louis, CV Mosby, 1982.

55. Goldberg S: Premature birth: Consequences for the parent-infant relationship. *Am Scientist* 67:214-220, 1979.

56. Trombly CA: Neurophysiological and developmental treatment approaches, in Trombly CA (ed): *Occupational Therapy for Physical Dysfunction,* ed 2. Baltimore, Williams & Wilkins, 1983.

57. Ayres AJ: *Sensory Integration and Learning Disorders.* Los Angeles, Western Psychological Services, 1972.

58. Montgomery P, Richter E: *Sensorimotor Integration for Developmentally Disabled Children: A Handbook.* Los Angeles, Western Psychological Services, 1978.

59. Morrison D, Pothier P, Horr K: *Sensory-Motor Dysfunction and Therapy in Infancy and Early Childhood.* Springfield, IL, Charles C Thomas, 1978.

60. Ottenbacher K, Short MA: Sensory integrative dysfunction in children: A review of theory and treatment, in Wolrich ML, Routh D (eds): *Advances in Developmental and Behavioral Pediatrics, vol 6.* Greenwich, CT, JAI Press, in press.

61. Prescott JW: Somatosensory deprivation and its relationship to the blind, in Jastrzembska ZS (ed): *The Effects of Blindness and Other Impairments on Early Development.* New York, American Foundation for the Blind, 1976.

62. Montagu A: *Touching,* ed 2. New York, Harper & Row, 1977.

63. Harlow HF, Suomi SJ: Nature of love—simplified. *Am Psychol* 25:162-168, 1970.

64. Mason WA, Berkson G: Effects of maternal mobility on the development of rocking and other behaviors in rhesus monkeys: A study with artificial mothers. *Dev Psychobiol* 8:197-211, 1975.

65. Gregg CL, Haffner ME, Korner AF: The relative efficacy of vestibular-proprioceptive stimulation and the upright position in enhancing visual pursuit in neonates. *Child Dev* 47:309-314, 1976.

66. Korner AF, Grobstein R: Visual alertness as related to soothing in neonates: Implications for maternal stimulation and early deprivation. *Child Dev* 37:867-876, 1966.

67. Freedman DG, Boverman H: The effects of kinesthetic stimulation on certain aspects of development in premature infants. *J Orthopsychiatry* 36:223-224, 1966.

68. Kramer M, Chamorro I, Green D et al.: Extra tactile stimulation of the premature infant. *Nurs Res* 24:324-334, 1975.

69. Neal MV: Vestibular stimulation and developmental behavior of the small premature infant. *Nurs Res Rep* 3:3-5, 1968.

70. Rice RD: Premature infants respond to sensory stimulation. *American Psychological Association Monitor* Nov. 8-9, 1975.

71. Ottenbacher K: Developmental implications of clinically applied vestibular stimulation: A review. *Phys Ther* 63:338-342, 1983.

72. Cohen EA, Lidsky K, Eyler F, et al.: Considerations during intervention with premature infants. *Developmental Disabilities Special Interest Section Newsletter.* American Occupational Therapy Association, 6:1-2, 1983.

73. Pederson DR, Ter Vrugt D: The influence of amplitude and frequency of vestibular stimulation on the activity of two-month-old infants. *Child Dev* 44:122-128, 1973.

74. Walsh RN: *Towards an Ecology of Brain.* New York, SP Medical and Scientific Books, 1981.

75. Bower TJR: *A Primer of Infant Development.* San Francisco, WH Freeman, 1977.

76. Lipsitt LP: Sensory and learning processes of newborns: Implications for behavioral disabilities, *Allied Health Behav Sci.* 1:493-522, 1978.

77. McClusky KA: The infant as organizer: Future directions in perceptual development, in Bloom K (ed): *Prospective Issues in Infancy Research.* Hillsdale NJ, Lawrence Erlbaum, 1981.

78. Papousek H, Papousek M: How human is the human newborn, and what else is to be done?, in Bloom K (ed): *Prospective Issues in Infancy Research.* Hillsdale NJ, Lawrence Erlbaum, 1981.

79. Lynch G, Wells J: Neuroanatomical plasticity and behavioral adaptability, in Teyler T (ed): *Brain and Behavior.* Stanford, CT, Greylock, 1978.

80. Clarke AM, Clarke ADB: Early experience: Its limited effect upon later development, in Schaffer D, Dunn J (eds): *The First Year of Life, Psychological and Medical Implications of Early Experience.* New York, John Wiley, 1979.

81. Hayden AH: The implications of infant intervention research. *Allied Health Behav Sci.* 1: 583-597, 1978.

82. Horowitz FD: Intervention and its effects on early development: What model of development is appropriate?, in Turner RR, Reese HW (eds): *Life-span Developmental Psychology Intervention.* New York, Academic Press, 1980.

83. Bronfenbrenner U: Is early intervention effective: Facts and principles of early intervention: A summary, in Clarke AM, Clarke ADB (eds): *Early Experience. Myth and Evidence.* New York, The Free Press, 1976.

84. Soboloff HR: Early intervention—Fact or fiction? *Dev Med Child Neurol* 23:261-266, 1981.

85. Harlow HF, Mears C: *The Human Model: Primate Perspectives.* New York, John Wiley, 1979.

86. Barnard MU: Supportive nursing care for the mother and newborn who are separated from each other. *Maternal Child Nurs* Mar/Apr:107-110, 1976.

87. Beckwith L: Caregiver-infant interaction and the development of the high risk infant, in Tjossem TD (ed): *Intervention Strategies for High Risk Infants and Young Children.* Baltimore, University Park Press, 1976.

88. Clark AL: Recognizing discord between mother and child and changing it to harmony, *Maternal Child Nurs* Mar/Apr:100-106, 1976.

89. Crowley C, Lester P, Pennington S: Assessment tool for measuring maternal attachment behaviors, in McNall L, Galeener J (eds): *Current Practice in Obstetrics and Gynecologic Nursing.* St. Louis, CV Mosby, 1976.

90. Green JA, Gustafson GE, West MJ: Effects of infant development on mother-infant interactions. *Child Dev* 51:199-207, 1980.

91. Thomas EAC, Martin JA: Analyses of parent-infant interaction. *Psychol Rev* 83:141-156, 1983.

92. Crowe TK: Father involvement in early intervention programs. *Phys Occup Ther Pediatr* 1(3):35-46, 1981.

93. Appoloni T, Cooke TP: Integrated programming at the infant, toddler, and preschool levels, in Guralnick M (ed): *Early Intervention and the Integration of Handicapped and Non-Handicapped Children.* Baltimore, University Park Press, 1978.

94. Levine MD: Developmental assessment. Infant and preschool developmental screening, in Levine MD, Carey WB, Crocker AC et al. (eds): *Developmental-Behavioral Pediatrics.* Philadelphia, WB Saunders, 1983.

95. Beach FA, Jaynes JA: Effects of early experience upon the behavior of animals. *Psychol Bull* 51:239-263, 1954.

96. Henderson ND: Effects of early experience upon the behavior of animals: The second twenty-five years of research, in Simmel EC (ed): *Early Experiences and Early Behavior.* New York, Academic Press, 1980.

97. Senf GM: Some methodological considerations in the study of abnormal conditions, in Walsh RN, Greenough WT (eds): *Environments as Therapy for Brain Dysfunction.* New York, Plenum, 1976.

98. Shaffer D, Dunn J: Introduction, in Shaffer D, Dunn J (eds): *The First Year of Life Psychological and Medical Implications of Early Experience.* New York, John Wiley, 1979.

99. Richards MPM: Effects on development of medical interventions and the separation of newborns from their parents, in Shaffer D, Dunn J (eds): *The First Year of Life, Psychological and Medical Implication of Early Experience.* New York, John Wiley, 1979.

100. Newman LF: Social and sensory environment of low birth weight infants in a special care nursery. An anthropological investigation. *J Nerv Ment Dis* 169: 448-455, 1981.

101. Gottfried AW, Wallace-Lande P, Sherman-Brown S et al.: Physical and social environment of newborn infants in special care units. *Science* 214:673-675, 1981.

102. Ross EF: Review and critique of research on the use of tactile and kinesthetic stimulation with premature infants. *Phys Occup Ther Pediatr* 4(1):35-49, 1984.

103. Beckwith L: Caregiver-infant interaction as a focus for therapeutic intervention with human infants, in Walsh RN, Greenough WT (eds): *Environments as Therapy for Brain Dysfunction.* New York, Plenum, 1976.

104. Widmayer SM, Field TM: Effects of Brazelton demonstrations for mothers on the development of preterm infants. *Pediatrics* 67:711-714, 1981.

105. Metzl MN: Teaching parents a strategy for enhancing infant development. *Child Dev* 51: 583-586, 1980.

106. Christophersen ER: Methodological issues in behavioral and developmental pediatrics, in Levine MD, Carey WB, Crocker AC et al. (eds): *Developmental-Behavioral Pediatrics.* Philadelphia, WB Saunders, 1983.

107. Sellick KJ, Over R: Effects of vestibular stimulation on motor development of cerebral-palsied children. *Dev Med Child Neurol* 22:476-483, 1980.

108. Ottenbacher K: Power and non-significant research results. *Dev Med Child Neurol* 23: 663-664, 1981.

109. Ottenbacher K: Statistical power and research in occupational therapy. *Occup Ther J Res* 2:13-26, 1982.

110. Ottenbacher K: The significance of power and the power of significance: Recommendations for occupational therapy research. *Occup Ther J Res* 4:38-50, 1984.

111. Capute AJ: Cost effectiveness of early therapy for the developmentally disabled. *Am Acad for Cerebral Palsy Dev Med* 32:6-7, 1981.

112. Lerer RJ: An open letter to an occupational therapist. *J Learn Disabil* 14:4-5, 1981.

113. Jenkins JR, Fewell R, Harris SR: Comparison of sensory integrative theory and motor programming. *Am J Ment Defic* 2:221-224, 1983.

114. Jenkins JR, Sells CJ: Physical and occupational therapy: Effects related to treatment, frequency and motor delay. *J Learn Disabil* 17:89-95, 1984.

115. Reese HW, Overton WF: Models, methods and ethics of intervention, in Turner RR,

Reese HW (eds): *Life-Span Developmental Psychology. Intervention.* New York, Academic Press, 1980.

116. Packer M, Rosenblatt D: Issues in the study of social behaviour in the first week of life, in Shaffer D, Dunn J (eds): *The First Year of Life. Psychological and Medical Implications of Early Experience.* New York, John Wiley, 1979.

117. Garbarino J: *Children and Families in the Social Environment.* New York, Aldine, 1982.

118. Bronfenbrenner U: Toward an experimental ecology of human development. *Am Psychologist* July:513-531, 1977.

T - #0573 - 101024 - C0 - 212/152/9 - PB - 9780866564328 - Gloss Lamination